Once a Month

Katharina Dalton

Fontana

An Imprint of HarperCollinsPublishers

A FONTANA ORIGINAL

First issued in 1978 by Fontana
an imprint of HarperCollins Publishers,
77–85 Fulham Palace Road,
Hammersmith, London W6 8JB

This Fontana edition first issued 1991

9   8   7   6

Copyright © Katharina Dalton 1978, 1980, 1983, 1987, 1991

The Author asserts the moral right to be
identified as the author of this work

ISBN 0 00 637727 0

Phototypeset by Input Typesetting Ltd, London
Printed and bound in Great Britain by
HarperCollins Book Manufacturing, Glasgow

CONDITIONS OF SALE
This book is sold subject to the condition
that it shall not, by way of trade or otherwise,
be lent, re-sold, hired out or otherwise circulated
without the publisher's prior consent in any form of
binding or cover other than that in which it is
published and without a similar condition
including this condition being imposed
on the subsequent purchaser

Once a Month

Dr Katharina Dalton was educated at the Royal Masonic School and trained as a chiropodist at the London Foot Hospital, writing the textbook *Essentials of Chiropody* (now in its seventh edition) when she was only 21. When widowed in the war she started her medical training at the Royal Free Hospital while still practising chiropody in the evenings. She qualified in 1948 and entered general practice where, during the first two months, she identified and successfully treated six women suffering from premenstrually related asthma, epilepsy and migraine. For 23 years she continued in general practice researching premenstrual syndrome. This interest resulted in her writing with Raymond Greene the first paper in British medical literature on the premenstrual syndrome, published in 1953. Working in 1954 with premenstrual syndrome patients at University College Hospital, London, led to her establishing there the world's first and oldest premenstrual syndrome clinic, which she still maintains and where, in conjunction with her Harley Street practice, she continues her studies into premenstrual syndrome and other related illnesses. She has been awarded the Charles Oliver Hawthorn BMA prize for outstanding research in general practice on three occasions and has also been awarded the Upjohn Fellowship, the Charlotte Brown prize and the Cullen prize by the Royal Free Hospital and the British Migraine Association prize by the Royal College of General Practitioners, of which she was a founder member. In 1971 she became the first woman President of the General Practice Section of the Royal Society of Medicine. She is the author of *The Premenstrual Syndrome* (1964), *The Menstrual Cycle* (1969), *Premenstrual Syndrome and Progesterone Therapy* (1977, 2nd ed. 1984), *Depression after Childbirth* (1980), *PMS Illustrated* (1990) and *PMS Goes to Court* (1990). Her books have been translated into sixteen languages. She has lectured extensively at home and abroad to both medical and lay audiences and has made numerous radio and TV broadcasts. She was awarded the Fellowship of the Royal College of General Practitioners in 1982. Dr Dalton is married to a Unitarian minister and has four children and five grandchildren.

Contents

Figures

Preface

This book is dedicated to the thousands of women who have confided in me the most personal and intimate details of their lives and from whom I have learned so much.

I am deeply grateful for the help received from all my family. To Drs Maureen and Michael Dalton who have been my most severe critics; to Mrs Anita Dalton and Mrs Wendy Holton who have patiently typed, corrected and retyped the manuscript before it was ready for submission to the publishers; to my niece, Mrs Sherryl Machray, for the artwork; and most of all to my long-suffering husband, Rev. Tom Dalton, for his invaluable ghost-writing of the entire book.

Finally my acknowledgement to David Duff and Tandem Press for the excerpt from *Albert & Victoria* and the journal of the Royal College of General Practitioners for permission to reproduce Figure 11.

KATHARINA DALTON
1978

Preface to Third Edition

In 1954 speaking to the General Practice Section of the Royal Society of Medicine, I ended my paper with the words:

> 'The cost of progesterone therapy is high, but when this charge is weighed against the price in terms of human misery, suffering and injustice, it is seen as a justifiable expense opening up a new vista of medicine.'

That vista is still opening up and during the last few years considerable progress has been made in the appreciation and understanding of menstrual problems and their treatment by the caring professions and also by the general public.

At the symposium on Premenstrual Syndrome at the International Congress of Psychosomatic Obstetrics and Gynaecology held in Berlin in September 1980, it was agreed that the premenstrual syndrome was a hormonal disease; therefore it was more suited for study by international meetings of endocrinologists rather than by psychologists. Of course there will always be those who disagree and suggest other approaches, which is as it should be, provided they are talking about the same diagnosed disease and have tried the same treatments, comparing them with other treatments to find the most successful.

New issues have emerged, such as the legal implications and the feminist movement. The premenstrual syndrome should not be a feminist issue. It is a hormonal disease, which deserves sympathy and understanding and requires to be diagnosed and treated.

This edition has been widely revised in the light of the findings of the past four years and includes a new chapter on legal implications. It is as up to date as it is possible to be, in the hope that the disease will be more commonly recognized, correctly diagnosed and properly treated.

KATHARINA DALTON
1983

Preface to Fourth Edition

The need for a fourth edition is a clear indicator that the demand for authentic information on the premenstrual syndrome is in no way slowing down. Nor, regrettably, are the torrents of misinformation, false information, mythical treatments or armchair theories diminishing. Indeed, it is these outpourings that are creating the confusion and bewilderment, not merely among the unfortunate sufferers of premenstrual syndrome, but also among the public, social workers and kindred health professionals. This adds a greater urgency to the provision of a fourth edition based on the accumulated experience of more than 38 years' continuous work with this pernicious disease.

Since this book was first written in 1977 there have been considerable advances in our knowledge of a woman's reproductive processes, such as the realization that each woman's menstrual cycle follows her own individual pattern which can vary considerably from woman to woman and yet remain normal; an appreciation that hormones are multifunctional; and an understanding of their behaviour, their transport through the body and their interactions within the target cell. Of particular importance are the recognition of progesterone receptors in the midbrain and the value of an estimation of the binding capacity of sex hormone binding globulin (SHBG). But there is still much ignorance and many questions are waiting to be answered. More new knowledge on the subject is eagerly awaited to help in solving some of the remaining mysteries.

In this edition a new chapter, 'Clearing the Confusion', has been added to help the readers to recognize the authenticity of what they read and hear about premenstrual syndrome. It is also needed to explain the difficulty of trying to diagnose correctly premenstrual syndrome using conventional methods of diagnosis. There is new information in almost every chapter, although some have had more alterations than others.

'Nature knows no pause in progress and development and attaches her curse on all inaction.' Both aspects of Goethe's nineteenth-century quotation are to be found in the story of premenstrual syndrome. The ongoing progress and development is to be found in my many writings from 1953 to the present day and is reflected in the never-ending stream of women daily referred for diagnosis and treatment. The other side, Nature's curse, is experienced by those countless women whose premenstrual sufferings continue because of the unwillingness of practitioners to use effective progesterone treatment until they have proved its success in double blind placebo controlled trials. To some that may sound a reasonable excuse for inaction, but let us take a lesson from history. Among sailors on long sea voyages, scurvy was the major cause of mortality and morbidity until the sixteenth century, when the Dutch discovered the value of a diet containing citrus fruits with which to combat scurvy. Nevertheless, it was not until 1932 that vitamin C (ascorbic acid) was identified as the curative agent of scurvy. In those earlier years no one was prepared to wait three centuries until science found the evidence – 'the proof of the pudding was in the eating' – and consequently many thousands of lives were saved from the ravages of scurvy. Today the women suffering from premenstrual syndrome who have been properly treated with progesterone know how very effective it is. Do the others have to wait 300 years until we know the exact mechanism of its action or are they deserving of treatment now?

During the preparation of the amendments to this fourth edition that question has been alongside another one in the forefront of my mind: how can I encourage my colleagues to learn the necessary new skills to enable them to diagnose correctly and properly treat premenstrual syndrome? This book has been written in the firm belief that all who read it with an open and unprejudiced mind will be able to learn a great deal about premenstrual syndrome and the reason for its treatment with progesterone. They will also appreciate that it is a very real disease which can have extremely serious consequences for some of its sufferers, but a disease that has responded magnificently to progesterone treatment ever since it was first used in 1948.

It now remains for me to continue with my work of healing and to express my gratitude to all those patients who have taught me so much; also to the many colleagues who have contributed to the increase and development of my understanding of the endocrine involvement in the disease, particularly my daughter, Dr Maureen Dalton. These appreciations would not be complete without an acknowledgement of the invaluable contribution of my hardworking staff, especially Wendy Holton and Jane Rogers. As always, your thanks and mine must go to my husband, the Rev. Tom Dalton, for all his support and untiring determination to maintain the high standard of readability for your enlightenment and pleasure. Finally my acknowledgement to William Heinemann Medical Books Ltd for permission to reproduce Figures 7 and 8 from my book *Premenstrual Syndrome and Progesterone Therapy*.

KATHARINA DALTON
1987

Preface to Fifth Edition

This new edition is not only evidence of the success of this popular book on premenstrual syndrome, but is also an indication of the importance and value of the information it provides for recognizing, diagnosing and understanding premenstrual syndrome.

The high standard established in this book contains the knowledge gained in over forty years of daily consultations, diagnosis and treatment of a wide range of PMS patients from all corners of the earth with their differing severities, presentations and need for personalized individual tailoring of treatment. The knowledge gained from this work is enhanced by a continuous scrutiny of worldwide medical and scientific research on the subject, especially the work of animal biologists on progesterone receptors. Too many people see this work as of purely scientific interest, but, in fact, their findings are of considerable importance, providing a greater understanding of the little known, but vital, functions of progesterone, receptor sites and progesterone receptors. A full understanding of their work enables a doctor to make a larger contribution to the good health of the patient and all members of her family.

'The art of medicine is valuable to us because it is conducive to health, not because of its scientific interest,' so wrote Cicero in the pre-Christian era, which is, of course, justification for this new, carefully revised and up-to-date edition. Among those especially deserving of my thanks are the many sparring partners who, over meals or late into the night in England and across the Atlantic, have discussed and dissected new findings, theories and ideas. Foremost among them have been my family, with the Rev. Tom Dalton clarifying my thoughts and understanding the arguments put forward by Drs Michael and Maureen Dalton, Mrs Wendy Holton and Dr Niall MacKenzie, and who, as usual, has ensured that it is all very readable. The contributions of Dr Glenn Bair in Topeka and Dr Mary Cortner in Kansas City must not be forgotten. The index was prepared by my granddaughters, Jennifer and Sarah Holton. My thanks go to them all and also those unknown scientific workers who have given us so much food for thought.

KATHARINA DALTON
May 1990

Introduction

Once a month, with monotonous regularity, chaos is inflicted on over a million British homes as premenstrual tension and other menstrual problems recur time and time again with a demoralizing repetition. Wonderfully happy and often idyllic marriages and partnerships break up under the strain of trying to live in harmony with an unpredictably irrational, and often violent, woman suffering from premenstrual syndrome. In such a situation the man may decide that there is no future for a happy union and he runs away. Is anyone going to blame him? The man who feels duty-bound to stand by his partner and their children will have to face up to a hard time before learning to live with these disconcerting situations. It is important for all men to learn that the relationship is not doomed; because once the premenstrual syndrome has been recognized and correctly diagnosed, it can be successfully treated, and the happy, lovely woman he once knew can be restored to him. This book explains how these menstrual problems can be completely relieved with the proper treatment, just as the pains of childbirth are today universally treated with pain-relievers and anaesthetics.

It has also been written to help men to understand those capricious and temperamental changes of women, so that the image of woman as uncertain, fickle, changeable, moody and hard-to-please, may go, to be replaced with the recognition that all these features can be understood in terms of the ever-

changing ebb and flow of her menstrual hormones and the
hormonal changes which occur within the body's cells.

It was as long ago as 1948 that I came across my first case
of premenstrual asthma, which responded successfully to
treatment with progesterone. Before a month had passed a
further case of asthma, two of epilepsy and one of migraine
had been found: all were related to menstruation. However,
for the premenstrual syndrome to be properly appreciated it
must be recognized in all its full variety of presentations.
Following a television documentary on the subject which
showed only four presentations – an alcoholic, a baby-
batterer, a husband-beater and a neurotic – the hospital's
postbag was filled with letters which suggested that the programme had been an eye opener to many viewers, those
letters containing such comments as:

> 'It was such a relief to know that so many other women
> experience the very real and deep feelings of anger, hatred
> and depression that I feel at period times.'

> 'I'm just like that woman.'

> 'I never told anyone because I thought they would never
> believe me.'

It is hoped this book will open many more eyes, for it is
estimated that there are in Britain today a million women
with incapacitating monthly problems which can and should
be eased.

The first step is to bring the subject out into the open and
not to sweep it under the carpet. Menstruation should be a
subject that can be discussed as openly as sex: anywhere, by
anybody, not merely in the bedroom or doctor's surgery. We
still suffer from the utterly Victorian attitude in which our
heroines in novels never menstruate. Since the first edition
of this book in 1978, there has been a most productive opening up of the subject. Indeed PMS is now the accepted
abbreviation of the premenstrual syndrome and represents a

favourite topic for many women's journals – but even today it is not routinely accepted as a hormone disorder. If women themselves do not yet associate the changes in their body and psyche with the changes in menstrual hormones, how can one hope that men will be able to understand it? After all, men don't even experience it. There must be a general recognition of the physical and psychological changes in a woman which can occur like a flash of lightning before menstruation, and which are not due to personality inadequacies.

While accepting that fatalities from premenstrual syndrome or period pains are rare and the suffering is short-lived, ending with menstruation, nevertheless the suffering, unhappiness and social consequences of it are without limitation.

One gynaecologist ranks premenstrual syndrome as the commonest cause of marital breakdown. In a general practice survey in England 75% of a sample of 521 women complained of at least one premenstrual symptom. In Britain the rate of attempted suicide shows that there is a sevenfold increase in the second half of the menstrual cycle compared with the pre-ovulatory half. Shoplifting is thirty times commoner in the second half of the cycle. As long ago as 1977 it was found that of 132 women who were currently under the care of the Premenstrual Syndrome Clinic at University College Hospital, London, 37% had a previous mental hospital admission; 34% had attempted suicide or homicide; 9% had alcoholic bouts; 6% were referred because of baby-battering and a further 4% sought treatment because of a fear of their injuries to their children becoming public knowledge; 6% had a history of criminal behaviour, such as smashing the windows of the Social Services headquarters, assaulting police or neighbours; 7% had premenstrual epilepsy and 5% had premenstrual asthma.

These are no trivialities, but are of vital concern to the patient, her family, society, and even the nation. This is shown in *Albert and Victoria*, David Duff's book on the married life of Queen Victoria (Muller, 1972). The following is an extract:

One of the reasons why Victoria continued to bear children was her belief that, by doing so, she kept her grip on Albert . . . When she was pregnant he was always kind, thoughtful, attentive of her every wish. Here was a problem that he could understand, a train of events to which he could attend. But he knew nothing of the imponderable in women. He was completely inexperienced. He did not appreciate the unreasoned emotions which surged like a maelstrom in Victoria's brain. Albert's answer to all the problems of life was to exercise reason . . . When Victoria began throwing things and screaming her accusations into his face, he would retire to write a paper on the cause of the outburst. She would then receive a letter beginning 'Dear Child' and containing simple ingredients for an antidote to emotion. This did not help matters. Albert soon learned that any action that he took at such times was wrong. Answering back led to faster, louder vituperation. Remaining quiet was classified as insulting. Retiring behind a locked door eventually led to an attack upon its panels by royal fists . . . Even [Lord] Melbourne, a pastmaster at dealing with women, had on one occasion quavered and feared to sit down as the fire blazed in the eyes of the eighteen-year-old queen. A Cabinet minister was known to fly from her presence, too frightened to follow the rule of withdrawal. Thus Albert looked forward to the period of pregnancy – it gave emotion a reason.

Prince Albert, Lord Melbourne and the Cabinet ministers were not as fortunately placed to deal with the premenstrual syndrome as you will be when you have read this book.

The premenstrual syndrome knows no geographical, social, racial or economic boundaries. Its sufferings and tragedies are spread evenly throughout our society. For many it is sufficient reassurance to know that other normal women also experience the same monthly feelings; while the knowledge that there is a satisfactory answer provides them with hope for the future.

1

The Curse of Eve

Once a month women are reminded that their reproductive system is still in the process of evolution. But it is no good waiting another two or three million years for Mother Nature to iron out the flaws. In the short term it is better to try to understand the way our body works, the problems with which the silent majority tries to cope and how best they can be helped.

The other natural functions of the body, such as growth, respiration, digestion and excretion go on day by day without pain. Indeed if pain is present it is abnormal, a cause for concern, and a thorough search is made to find and eradicate the disease. On the other hand the two natural feminine physiological processes, menstruation and childbirth, are seldom completely without pain. It is thought that less than one woman in ten goes through her childbearing years without at some time suffering from period pain or premenstrual tension. It is now universally accepted (although it was not always so) that women experiencing pain during labour are deserving of relief with analgesics and anaesthetics, and they even go into training for this one-day event with weekly relaxation classes. One hopes that the days of enlightenment are not too far off when treatment for the relief of period pains and premenstrual problems will be accepted as the natural right of every woman the world over.

Menstruation represents a failed pregnancy, and only

occurs if the woman is neither pregnant nor breast feeding. It was therefore a comparative rarity in primitive society. A normal woman could expect to menstruate once a month for an average of 35 years, but our greatgrandmothers, who breastfed their families of twelve children as the only known method of contraception, averaged only 11 years of intermittent menstruation. By contrast, today's mother of two, who breastfeeds for an average of three months, may expect almost continuous menstrual cycles for 33 years.

> ANNE, 34 years, was brought to the surgery by the Catholic priest, because of a severe asthma attack which accompanied her last menstruation. She was then asked if asthma had also accompanied her previous menstruation before this last one. She took a few minutes to think about it before admitting, 'I was only eighteen at the time and I can't really remember.' She had fourteen children, and for the last sixteen years had either been pregnant or breast feeding.

Pain is not the only symptom associated with menstruation: there are also those psychological and bodily symptoms which come out of the blue once a month, usually just before menstruation, and come under the omnibus heading of the Premenstrual Syndrome. Such examples include Barbara and Carol.

BARBARA wrote:

> 'I have such drastic changes in personality before a period I think I am going mad. I cannot understand how I can feel so differently towards my children, one day loving and caring for them and the next day hateful and rough, so bad-tempered and smacking them for nothing. How guilty I feel when I see my own daughter, aged five, copying me and smacking her dolls.'

CAROL wrote:

> 'I have one fantastic week each month, but after ovulation

*my whole body changes, my breasts start to swell, I look
five months pregnant with a swollen tummy, my chest is
tight and I just can't breathe because of asthma. There is
usually a migraine on the first day of menstruation.'*

Relief is possible for women with painful periods and also
those with premenstrual symptoms, like Barbara and Carol.
However, first it is necessary for them to make the connection
between their symptoms and menstruation, which means it
depends either on the patient herself recognizing it, or her
husband, mother or close friend, or her doctor. Once the
problem is recognized, treatment is available, as will be seen
in later chapters.

It has been said 'Man is born to suffer, but woman is born
to suffer more' and sometimes it seems that no efforts are
being made to ease a woman's sufferings. Consider this list
of excuses culled from recent letters:

'It's not fatal and doesn't last long.'

'She'll get over it.'

'Cool it, lady, you're neurotic.'

*'Things will be easier when you're married/or had
children/or the children have grown up.'*

'Learn to live with it and take more exercise.'

*'Accept the symptoms – you're not going mad – and learn
to relax.'*

'Only because you've not enough to do' (three children
all under school age).

'You're working too hard' (one child at school).

*'You're only trying to jump on the bandwagon like 90%
of other women.'*

And so the excuses go on with the adoption of an ostrich-like attitude to once-a-month problems and no efforts made to solve them.

There is nothing new about these menstrual problems; even Hippocrates, the father of medicine, blamed premenstrual tension on 'the agitated blood of a woman seeking a way of escape from the womb'. Primitive man found it difficult to understand how women could lose blood month by month, yet neither be ill nor die. Even today many men are amazed that women can accept the regular loss of blood so cheerfully, when they themselves panic each time their nose bleeds or they cut a finger. But it is only rarely that women complain of the blood itself – it is how they feel and look, and the pains they suffer, that worries them. When primitive tribes lived in isolation there might be only one menstruating woman present at any one time. It was natural then to endow her with supernatural powers, normally ascribed to their gods. These powers included her ability to stop hailstorms, whirlwinds and lightning if she went out into the open unclothed. Menstrual blood was also thought to be endowed with valuable properties, such as being able to extinguish fires, temper metals and fashion swords as well as protecting man against wounds in battle. A thread soaked in menstrual blood was considered a valuable treatment for epilepsy and headache (today we often find that once menstruation starts, the premenstrual epilepsy or headache is relieved).

Myths about menstruation are worldwide. In some parts of the world the presence of a menstruating woman was believed to be able to sour wines, blight crops, rust iron or bronze and turn copper green. She could cause cattle to abort, seeds to dry up, fruit on trees to die, bright mirrors to become dulled, the edge to be taken off sharpened metal, a hive of bees to perish, the strings of harps to break, clocks to stop and linen to turn black. Can one wonder that women in India went into Purdah at these times?

During the Middle Ages it was believed that menstruation demonstrated the essential sinfulness and inferiority of women, who were therefore forbidden to attend church or take communion, a custom still continued in the Greek Orthodox Church today. For this reason also, Orthodox Jewish women are instructed to make themselves plain and unattractive during menstruation to avoid exciting their husbands sexually. Following menstruation, the woman is required to undergo a ritualistic cleansing by immersing herself three times in a 'body of water'.

In different countries there are many local customs associated with menstruation, which are concerned chiefly with the local industries and fear of their failure. In Indonesia, menstruating women may not enter tobacco fields or work in rice paddies. In Saigon they may not be employed in opium factories, lest the opium burns bitter. In France and Germany they were excluded from wineries and breweries lest they turned the wine or beer sour; and in the Canary Islands today, women are not allowed in the grape-crushing area. In France, the presence of a menstruating woman during the boiling process in sugar refineries might turn the sugar black. Parsees in India may not look at a fire lest their glance extinguishes it. In Syria, if pickling is done by menstruating women it will cause the food to putrefy. In South Africa, menstruating women may not come into contact with cattle for fear the milk will turn sour. Until the last century in England it was believed that if menstruating women salted meat it would not keep.

The problems associated with menstruation are obviously not new, they represent the eternal mystery of woman, but what is new is the changing attitude of the medical profession which now contains a few doctors, far too few, who have interested themselves in these problems and have shown that they can be successfully treated, and treated without witchcraft. Other doctors are trying to learn how to correctly diagnose and properly treat these problems, but are often confused by the bewildering amount of misinformation and, far too often, wrong information that is constantly being presented to them by those with little or no practical experience of premenstrual syndrome, or by entrepreneurs looking for financial gain. These doctors see this shamefully neglected subject of menstruation, with its complexity of symptoms which can change a woman from Jekyll to Hyde within minutes, as a challenge to be met.

The Menstrual Cycle

To ensure the continuation of the human species, nature has evolved, in a woman, a system which produces an egg cell at precisely the right time for it to be fertilized by the sperm of the male. Research has shown that this is not the simple process we used to believe, it is really very complex. There is no need for us to go into all the details, for nature's basic system is the menstrual cycle which can be explained in quite simple terms and still be a correct account of the process of childbearing.

Woman is born with two ovaries containing thousands of immature egg cells. Each month, in response to a message from the pituitary gland, one of the unripe egg cells develops inside a tiny microscopic ring of cells, which gradually increases to form a little balloon or cyst called the Graafian follicle. These cells make the menstrual hormone, *oestrogen*, about which we will be hearing much more in later pages. When the little egg cell is fully developed, it appears as a blister on the surface of the ovary and receiving a further message from the pituitary gland it bursts and releases the mature egg cell. When this occurs it is known as *ovulation*. The egg cell makes its way down the fallopian tubes to the womb, a journey that takes about fourteen days. Meanwhile, the yellow scar tissue left behind when the blister burst fills up with new cells which produce the second important menstrual hormone, *progesterone*. The progesterone acts on the lining of the womb to turn it into a soft spongy layer in which the fertilized egg cell can embed itself if a pregnancy occurs. During intercourse millions of male sperm are projected into the vagina and journey through the womb up into one of the fallopian tubes in an attempt to fertilize the egg cell so that conception will occur and pregnancy can begin. The fertilized egg passes into the womb and becomes embedded in the new, soft lining where it develops into a baby. In which case progesterone will continue to be produced to protect the developing baby from being rejected by the mother's womb.

However, if the egg cell has not been fertilized the production of progesterone begins to fall and about fourteen days after ovulation the soft, spongy lining of the womb, which is then not needed, disintegrates and is shed together with the unfertilized egg cell, as menstrual blood or *menstruation*. Thus menstruation is failed pregnancy.

We are All Different
Women are different in so many ways, size, shape, colouring, facial characteristics, personality, parentage, family size and position, environment, education, previous illnesses, reactions to food and to drugs, that it is no surprise to realize that women are also different in their menstrual pattern and how they react to menstrual symptoms.

Men are also different. The range of emotions shown by men to sufferers of premenstrual syndrome and menstrual problems covers a wide span from genuine sympathy and understanding to annoyance, amazement, anger, aggression, disbelief, ridicule and withdrawal. There is even the partner who says, 'You've had it long enough, you ought to know how to deal with it.'

Normal Variations of Menstruation
Each woman's menstrual cycle is unique and individually her own, so there are considerable variations. The menstrual flow, which is the disintegrated lining of the womb, may appear as a pink watery discharge, as thick red blood or be reddish brown or black, and may contain shreds or small blood clots. All these variations are normal and healthy. Similarly, menstruation may occur every 21 or every 36 days, or anywhere in between, and it will still be considered as normal and compatible with full reproductive function. A

variation in the length of cycle of four days month by month is also normal and almost to be expected. Ovulation occurs no earlier than 14 days before menstruation so, taking into account the different lengths of menstrual cycles, ovulation can occur as early as day 10 in a 21-day cycle or as late as day 22 in a 36-day cycle.

This variation in the length of menstrual cycle is also important in determining the timing of medication for menstrual problems. Some treatments for premenstrual syndrome suggest starting on day 12 and continuing until day 26, but this is of little value to the woman with a 36-day cycle, who then receives no medication during the vital last ten days of her cycle. From all this it is obvious that there can be no standard dose, or timing, of treatment, which will be appropriate to every woman suffering from premenstrual syndrome. Each woman requires an individual regime of treatment for success.

There are also variations in the amount of menstrual flow on different days of menstruation. Some women have the heaviest flow on the first, second and third day and then stop abruptly. Others have moderate loss for a day or two and then the heaviest loss on the third or fourth day. Then there are those women who merely have a scanty loss for a day or two before the flow gradually increases in amount. It is important for the doctor to know which is the day of heaviest loss because, in premenstrual syndrome, the spontaneous relief of symptoms will not occur until the day of heaviest loss, so for some women symptoms may occur during the early days of menstruation.

Phases of the Menstrual Cycle
Menstrual cycles vary considerably in length in different women, but for the purpose of understanding the hormonal changes in the menstrual cycle it is convenient to divide it up into seven phases of four days each, which assumes the woman has a precise cycle of 28 days. It will be noticed that

in the seven phases there are no two phases which have the same levels of hormones circulating in the blood (Fig. 1).

The phases are:

Days 1–4   *Menstruation* with rising oestrogen levels

Days 5–8   *Postmenstruum* with peak oestrogen levels

Days 9–12   *Late postmenstruum* with falling oestrogen levels

Days 13–16 *Ovulation* with low oestrogen and peak levels of follicle stimulating hormones (FSH) and luteinizing hormones (LH)

Days 17–20 *Post-ovulation* with rising oestrogen and progesterone levels

Days 21–24 *Early premenstruum*. Peak oestrogen and progesterone levels

Days 25–28 *Premenstruum*. Falling levels of oestrogen and progesterone.

The first four days of menstruation and the last four before menstruation are known as the *paramenstruum*; it is a useful term which is used in surveys, for these days occur regardless of the length of a woman's cycle. Any adjustment due to a cycle length longer or shorter than 28 days is made in the last postmenstruum. In long cycles the postmenstruum may be eight days more, while short cycles will have a short postmenstruum. For comparison the daily levels of male hormones are steady day by day, as shown in Fig. 2.

The attitudes of women to regular menstruation vary considerably. Some think of it as a sign of normality and an indication of good health. Others regard it as a sign of femininity with maternal attributes, or it may be just an assurance that the woman is not pregnant now, but is fertile. Menopausal women see menstruation as a sign of their youthfulness to which they are so anxious to cling, whilst those who see menstruation as a once-a-month nuisance to be tolerated as Mother Nature's wish, wonder why medical scientists have not given more thought to the abolition of the associated ailments and complaints.

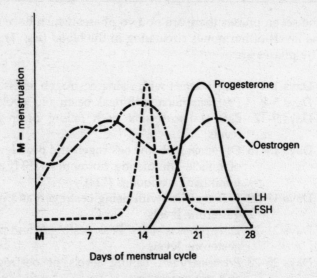

Fig. 1 Menstrual hormone variations during the menstrual cycle

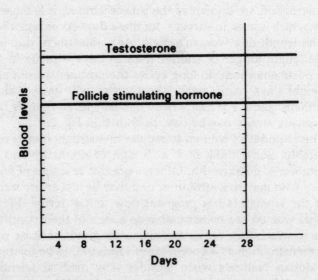

Fig. 2 Male hormone levels during a month

A study of the words used colloquially throughout the world to describe menstruation is fascinating. In Britain, Egypt and Mexico words are used to imply a state of ill-health or pain, such as 'being unwell' or 'having the blues'. In Yugoslavia, Mexico, Egypt and the Philippines the menstrual bleeding is often personified as a 'visitor', also in Britain it may be 'the curse' or given the familiarity of an old friend like 'Charlie' or 'Archie'. In Nigeria and Jamaica young girls are taught about 'growing up' using the analogy of 'flowers and bees' so that when menstruation occurs it is called 'flowers'. Women in Egypt and Korea use terms associated with sanitary towels and bathing. In Indonesia the words used are associated with pollution or with purification. In the Philippines the phrase 'desire for abortion' is sometimes used when describing menstruation.

Psychologists object to the use of the word 'curse', claiming that it conditions women to expect trouble with menstruation. On the other hand women have as many menstrual problems in Nigeria and Jamaica where terms with more favourable associations are used. There is no doubt that psychological factors do play a part in menstrual problems, but this is only secondary to the hormonal effects.

2

Mood Swings

'Tell me, Doctor, why does my wonderful wife, with her perfect figure and lovely nature, suddenly spit with rage for no obvious reason once a month?'

There are innumerable answers to that question. Most likely the blame will be laid on external events, while the upset of chemicals which occurs within her body at the time of menstruation will be overlooked. These chemical changes can produce changes in personality or sudden swings of mood, as menstruation approaches, followed by a return to normality as or after the menstrual flow starts. This is known as premenstrual syndrome (or more familiarly as PMS). Doctors use the word 'Syndrome' for a group of complaints or symptoms which come together.

The mood swings may vary from a minor nuisance to a major catastrophe. There may be an unexpected reaction to a trivial irritation, a hilarious conversation abruptly ended by a cutting or sarcastic remark, a blunt rebuke or just a loss of a sense of humour. On the other end of the scale there may be violent verbal abuse or smashing of things and throwing the nearest object; at the far extreme lies the possibility of suicide, homicide or infanticide. It is easy for an observer to attribute this to a lack of self-control, a mere temperamental outburst or even evidence of the woman's true character. Too rarely are these mood swings attributed to the natural ebb and flow of the menstrual hormones over which the woman has such little control.

These premenstrual mood swings are widespread and occur in at least half of all women. But this does mean that there is also another 50% of women who do not experience them at all and do not know what the other half are suffering. Why this fortunate 50% do not suffer is explained in Chapter 17. Men do not experience such changes in hormone levels. The male sex hormones, or chemical messengers, are on an even keel day by day throughout the month, as shown by the levels of follicle stimulating hormone (FSH) and testosterone in Fig. 2. How different are the levels of the woman's four sex hormones, follicle stimulating hormone (FSH), luteinizing hormone (LH), oestrogen and progesterone which vary day by day throughout the month as shown in Fig. 1. Only a slight imbalance in any of these levels is enough to cause problems for a woman.

'Premenstrual Syndrome' is used to embrace *any symptoms or complaints which regularly come just before or during early menstruation but are absent at other times of the cycle.* It is a precise definition and means that the symptoms must be present each and every month. Symptoms must occur premenstrually and there must be a symptom-free phase each cycle. It is the absence of symptoms after menstruation which is so important in this definition.

There are some 150 different symptoms which can be included in this syndrome such as tension, depression, tiredness, irritability, backache, asthma, sinusitis, epilepsy and gain in weight but, fortunately, no woman suffers from *all* the possible symptoms. All these individual symptoms can also be experienced by men, but in the male they are random occurrences, not occurring once every month. It is only in women that we find these symptoms occurring cyclically and regularly related to menstruation.

Premenstrual syndrome needs to be differentiated from menstrual distress. *Menstrual distress covers symptoms present throughout the menstrual cycle with increased intensity before or during menstruation.* Such symptoms may be intermittent as with headaches, or continuously present day by day as with anxiety and depression. It is unfortunately true that in all chronic diseases (for instance, rheumatoid arthritis, bronchitis, multiple sclerosis, schizophrenia, glaucoma), women find their symptoms increase before menstruation.

Most sufferers of the premenstrual syndrome suffer from more than one symptom at the same time. For instance, many sufferers will notice weight-gain and increased tension before the onset of a premenstrual headache. The removal of only one symptom, for example by giving a tranquillizer to ease the tension, will be of little help to the gain in weight and the headache.

It is also important to remember that the definition of premenstrual syndrome requires not only the presence of symptoms related to menstruation, but also the complete absence of these symptoms at other times of the menstrual cycle. It is this absence of symptoms and the change of mood after menstruation back to being a happy, energetic, vivacious woman once more, which clinches the diagnosis.

This letter from a patient illustrates the point:

> 'I have suffered from the usual premenstrual symptoms for five years and my tension, irritability and depression were put down to nerves, but I must say I could never understand this as it was only at certain times of the month that I seemed to be so nervy, tense and unconfident and depressed. I found that about ten to twelve days before my period it was as if something was draining out of me and as if something chemical was happening, and so often I tried to pull myself together at this time and it just never worked. I get so irritable and nervy a week before that I just want to shut myself up in the house and I feel as if I can't go to work and socially I avoid any sort of engagement at this time of the month. At other times I'm OK.'

The exact type and severity of symptoms varies with each individual, but in every sufferer her own time-schedule of discomfort is the same, month by month, or rather, cycle by cycle. The easiest tool for recognizing the relationship of symptoms to menstruation and the absence of symptoms at other times of the cycle is the simple menstrual chart discussed fully in Chapter 3. This is widely used by doctors, and it is easy enough for anyone to copy one for themselves.

The start of the mood swings may be quite sudden and the victim may even surprise herself by her own outrageous behaviour. It has been described as 'a blanket of fog which enfolds me', while a 20-year-old student thought of it as 'changing from top gear to bottom in the car'. In other cases, the beginning may be quite gradual, symptoms becoming worse day by day. Problems may start at ovulation and last the full fourteen days until menstruation, so that one sufferer felt she was 'crazy for half my life', or it may last for only days or hours before the onset of menstruation. Even if it only lasts for a matter of days it can still be a great source of concern, as one letter-writer described:

> 'Every month it is the same and the thought of being knocked out for a couple of days each month for the next twenty or so years fills me with a sense of desperation as it is such a waste of days which could be used for living instead of for wallowing in.'

Indeed in premenstrual epilepsy the attack may be measured in minutes or hours rather than in days before menstruation, however long or short the menstrual cycle may be. The symptoms tend to last longer as one approaches the menopause. A 42-year-old teacher wondered if 'this gradual lengthening of the negative mood would mean that there may soon be a time when there is no bright spell left at all'. It was good to be able to reassure her that however long the premenstrual mood lasted, there would always be a bright spell once a month after menstruation, for premenstrual symptoms do not start earlier than fourteen days before menstruation, however long or short the menstrual cycle may be.

For many women the onset of menstruation works like a charm, and as the blood flows the relief has been likened to 'a cloud lifting' or 'the curtain opens again'. The very occasional sufferer may even be freed from her symptoms a day or just a few hours before menstruation starts. Yet others may find relief is slower. The relief of symptoms comes with the full menstrual flow, so that those women who find that at the beginning there is only slight spotting of blood for one, two or more days, will not get relief of symptoms until the spotting changes to a full menstrual flow. Indeed, their worst days may be during those early days of spotting and they may not regain their joy of living until a couple of days after menstruation has finished. When it's over, one may hear a loving husband announce, 'She's now like the girl I married!'

It is often the outside observer who notices the mood swings first, usually the husband or mother, but occasionally an employer, social worker, friend or daughter. Following a television feature called *Pull Yourself Together, Woman*, one husband wrote:

> '*I was so startled to recognize in all these cases the symptoms from which my wife has been suffering for the past eight years. The connection with the menstrual cycle may seem less direct but nevertheless the symptoms are heightened in the premenstrual period and she is free of them thereafter. Briefly they include acute anxiety and depression (in any order as it seems impossible to distinguish cause and effect) manifested by physical symptoms of pressure on the head (variously described as an iron band around the head or a heavy weight at the top of the head) and giddiness; and by psychological symptoms such as agoraphobia, panic, guilt, obsessions and depressions, sometimes to the extent of suicidal notions.*'

Women in their mid-thirties may have been married, been on the pill and stopped; they have had their pregnancies and possibly been sterilized. All these are factors which increase the incidence and severity of premenstrual syndrome. It was noted at the International Symposium on Premenstrual Syndrome held in South Carolina in 1983 that when introducing their papers on different aspects of their work, the many speakers described the age of the patients they had studied, and these were invariably in their mid-thirties. They described women who had attended Premenstrual Syndrome Clinics and had been diagnosed as suffering from the disease. But all too often it is the young adolescents and those in their early twenties who suffer in silence without being diagnosed; they are thought to be bad tempered, miserable and lazy; they are unloved and so end up in bad company, leading to yet more problems. The title 'Mid-Thirty Syndrome' fortunately never caught on and one hopes it will be forgotten. It is unfair to those in other age groups.

Fortunately there is an end to this exclusively feminine syndrome, in that when the menopausal changes are complete, menstruation ends and so do the monthly fluctuations of mood and other symptoms. This is the time when one may look forward to the era of serenity. Menopause marks the end of childbearing, ovulation ceases and gradually women's hormones readjust.

Clearing the Confusion

Without a doubt there is much confusion about premenstrual syndrome. The medical profession is confounded by it, no matter whether they are gynaecologists, psychiatrists or endocrinologists; even general practitioners, who see the condition first and are in an ideal situation for treating it, are perplexed. Few consultants know anything about it, even though premenstrual syndrome invades every speciality. Add to this the appalling ignorance and utter befuddlement of the media presentation on the subject and it is only too easy to understand how the bewilderment continues to grow. It is hoped that this chapter will clear away these mists of confusion.

In such a situation it is essential to establish a definition of the disease in question in order to achieve a diagnosis of the disease. The definition of premenstrual syndrome is *'the presence of any symptoms or complaints which regularly come just before or during early menstruation but are absent at other times of the cycle'*. The precise definition means that three requirements must be fulfilled for a correct diagnosis:

- 1 Symptoms must be present every month for at least the previous three months.
- 2 Symptoms must be present premenstrually, and cannot start before ovulation.

- 3 There must be complete absence of symptoms after menstruation for a minimum of seven days.

The successful treatment of any disease depends on the accuracy of the diagnosis. To achieve that accuracy a time-honoured method of diagnosis has been developed. This is by consideration of symptoms, signs and investigations. That means the doctor listens to the patient's account of the complaint, takes note of any signs of disease which may be revealed by examination, and studies the result of blood tests, X-rays and other investigations. The doctor accepts the patient's account of her symptoms (be they a sore throat or a pain in some part of the body), and having examined for signs and considered the results of tests he makes his diagnosis and treats appropriately. When women come to their doctor claiming that they have premenstrual symptoms the doctor all too often accepts their claim at face value without appreciating the need to further check the diagnosis before treating.

Time Relationship of Symptoms to Menstruation

With premenstrual syndrome the doctor must verify the diagnosis, for there are no special symptoms indicative of the disease: all the symptoms can be complained of by men, children and postmenopausal women, none of whom menstruate. The disease only affects women of childbearing age. There are no specific signs discovered on examination and no definitive investigations. How, then, can an accurate diagnosis be made in a disease which has no special symptoms, no specific signs and no distinctive investigations? There is, however, a diagnostic clue in the time relationship of symptoms to menstruation. It therefore becomes necessary to find a new method of diagnosis which will enable this relationship to be clearly established.

Psychiatrists use questionnaires in their diagnosis of disease, asking the patient numerous questions and analysing the replies. This is a useful method, enabling numerical scores to be obtained for an individual's level of, for instance, depression, anxiety, neuroticism, or marital stability. This score can then be used to compare the results of different treatments, but not for diagnosing premenstrual syndrome.

Menstrual Distress Questionnaires

In 1968 Rudolph Moos designed a questionnaire which is most effective in demonstrating the amount of distress caused by menstruation, although it cannot differentiate premenstrual syndrome from menstrual pain or distress. The Moos Menstrual Distress Questionnaire has been used in some trials of the syndrome, in which the woman is asked to complete 47 different questions each night on a six-point scale. This includes questions such as: 'Today did you have any orderliness? . . . excitement? . . . loneliness?' It is a method which relies on the honesty, reliability and obsession of the candidate. While it is easy to complete the questionnaire and carefully consider your reply for one, or even seven consecutive days, one doubts the accuracy of the method when, as in Sampson's trials in 1978 and 1988 women completed the questionnaire every single day for six months. There is always a need for caution in interpreting the results of questionnaires when they are used for purposes other than those for which they were designed.

Unfortunately, these questionnaires concentrate on common psychiatric symptoms and do not cover all the 150 possible symptoms which may occur in premenstrual syndrome. Useful missing questions would include: 'Did you shoplift today?' 'Did you have too much alcohol today?' 'How many puffs of your inhaler did you need to control your asthma?' 'Could you wear your contact lenses today?' Furthermore, the questionnaires cannot be answered by those few severely ill patients who are temporarily confused, deluded or hallucinated during the premenstruum, but are free of symptoms during the postmenstruum.

It must not be forgotten that the information obtained from questionnaires needs to be prospective, obtained daily, rather than retrospectively by such questions as: 'During the days before menstruation do you suffer from . . . ?' Today women have been educated by the media to know that headaches, bloatedness, backache and irritability tend to occur premenstrually, so if they suffer from such symptoms at all they will automatically assume that their headache or other symptom occurs before menstruation.

The Menstrual Chart

If one is to rely on the help of the patient in making the diagnosis, it is important to avoid subjecting her to unnecessary strain in order to eliminate the possibility of inaccuracy and guesswork. The menstrual chart shown in Fig. 3 is widely used by doctors, and it is easy enough for anyone to copy out for themselves.

The purpose of the chart is to provide the precise information necessary to ensure that an accurate diagnosis of premenstrual syndrome can be made, by recording the actual dates of menstruation and the days when symptoms or complaints are present. The woman is asked to choose only her three most important symptoms, those complaints she would most like to lose. These are then given symbols, such as 'H' for headache, 'X' for quarrels, 'T' for tension. A small letter, 'h', 'x' or 't', can be used for mild symptoms and the capital for when they are really severe. There is never a need to use more than one letter for any one symptom. 'M' may be used to represent menstruation, although some use 'P' for period (it matters not at all what symbols are used). The woman is then asked to complete the menstrual chart each night in relation to whether the symptom was present or absent and whether it was severe during that day. Some women like to insert a dot on those days when they feel well; this ensures that they complete it each night. It should be completed daily regardless of the phase of the menstrual cycle or the apparent cause of the symptom. Doctors interpreting the chart are fully aware that there may be other circumstances which cause the same symptoms – for instance, spending several

Name _____ Year _____

	Jan.	Feb.	Mar.	Apr.	May	Jun.	Jul.	Aug.	Sep.	Oct.	Nov.	Dec.
1												
2												
3												
4												
5												
6												
7												
8												
9												
10												
11												
12												
13												
14												
15												
16												
17												
18												
19												
20												
21												
22												
23												
24												
25												
26												
27												
28												
29												
30												
31												

Fig. 3 Menstrual chart

hours at the hospital while your son is having his lacerated leg sutured by the casualty officer may well cause you to feel tense, irritable or depressed, regardless of the phase of the cycle. Again, you may well feel exhausted or have a headache after an all-night delay of your flight coming back from holiday.

By using a menstrual chart it becomes immediately obvious whether symptoms are clustered around menstruation, as in Fig. 4, or occurring haphazardly throughout the month, as in Fig. 5. It is easy to see the duration of menstruation or of symptoms.

If the menstrual cycle is short the 'M's will be going up the chart; if it is long the 'M's go down the chart. Furthermore, it is not necessary for the woman to be menstruating to obtain information as to the cyclical character of her symptoms. Cyclical symptoms can occur at times of the occasional missed menstruation and also before menstruation has begun; at the menopause or after removal of the womb or ovaries.

One mother, a sales executive, who was herself receiving treatment for premenstrual syndrome, was disturbed to find that her well-behaved daughter of thirteen had occasional 'off' days when she would be rude and lazy, which was out of character for her. Then the mother received reports from school that her daughter had occasional rebellious days during which she found it hard to accept discipline but easy to be rude. The mother carefully recorded the dates of her outbursts, which are shown on the chart in Fig. 6, with outbursts occurring at intervals of 32 to 36 days. When later the daughter started to menstruate, the timing of her menstrual cycle averaged 35 days. In fact, this mother had diagnosed premenstrual syndrome before menstruation had started. It is not necessary for menstruation or ovulation to occur before the premenstrual syndrome develops.

If the chart does not appear to show a relationship of symptoms to menstruation, there is no point in trying to make it fit the PMS pattern. It is wiser to show the chart to your doctor, as it may contain valuable clues which will

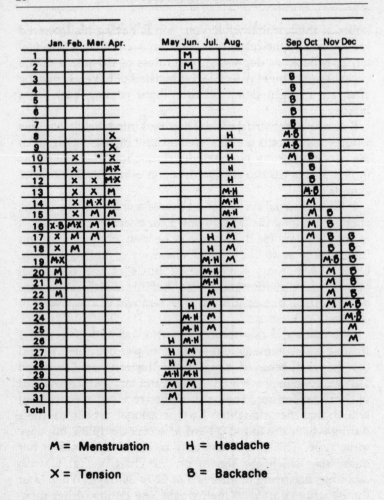

M = Menstruation   H = Headache

X = Tension   B = Backache

Fig. 4 Menstrual charts diagnostic of premenstrual syndrome

enable him or her to appreciate the true problem and treat you appropriately. It is not unknown for some women to copy a chart straight from the book and then ask for help. Unfortunately, in these circumstances there is little the doctor can do to help the sufferer.

	Jan.	Feb.	Mar.	Apr.		May	Jun.	Jul.	Aug.
1	X		X	M					H
2			X	M					
3			X	M		H	H		
4									
5				X					H
6				X		H		H	
7			M			H			
8	X		M·X				H		
9	X		M				H		
10		X	M				H		
11									H
12		M				M		H	
13		M	X	X		M			
14		M				M·H	H		
15		X				M		M	
16	X					M		M	
17	M					M		M	M
18	M					M	M	M	M
19	M	X				M	M	M	M
20		X		X				M	M
21			X					M	M
22			X			H	M		M
23	X					H	M		
24	X						M·H		
25	X								
26		X							
27				X					
28			X	M		H			H
29				M			H		
30	X			M				H	
31						H			
Total									

M = Menstruation   X = Quarrels

H = Headaches

Fig. 5 Menstrual chart with unrelated symptoms

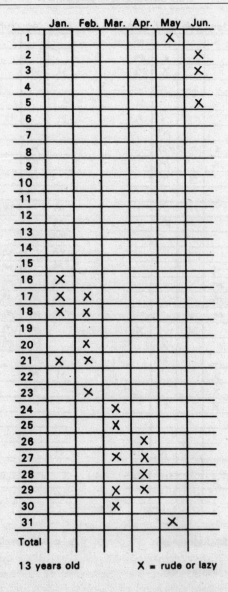

	Jan.	Feb.	Mar.	Apr.	May	Jun.
1					X	
2						X
3						X
4						
5						X
6						
7						
8						
9						
10						
11						
12						
13						
14						
15						
16	X					
17	X	X				
18	X	X				
19						
20		X				
21	X	X				
22						
23		X				
24			X			
25			X			
26				X		
27			X	X		
28				X		
29			X	X		
30			X			
31					X	
Total						

13 years old   X = rude or lazy

Fig. 6 Chart of adolescent girl with cyclical symptoms before start of menstruation

On rare occasions the diagnosis may be made by the observations of others which reveal the cyclical character of symptoms. For instance, a legal executive took note of the days on which her secretary's typing deteriorated and she became aggressive. When this revealed a pattern of every 30 to 33 days she advised her to seek medical help. The value of information received from police, prison officers and medical records is mentioned in Chapter 15.

The PMT-Cator is a sophisticated circular diagnostic chart developed by the PMT Clinic, Dulwich Hospital, London, and is useful as a screening tool in a busy clinic. The woman chooses five main symptoms to record daily, starting on the first day of menstruation and scoring each symptom from 0 (none) to 3 (severe). The chart is designed so that a disc covers all previous recordings, so that each night's entry will be unbiased. At the end of the cycle the woman can remove the top disc and add up her scores for the first seven days and the last seven days before menstruation. If the final score for the premenstrual week exceeds 25, or if the premenstrual score subtracted from the postmenstrual score exceeds 14, a probable diagnosis exists. A definitive diagnosis of premenstrual syndrome cannot be made from a single disc; many women have severe symptoms for only three or four days in the premenstruum and the presence of postmenstrual symptoms needs further investigation.

Hormone Blood Tests

Tests to determine the blood level of progesterone are of little value in the diagnosis of premenstrual syndrome, as the secretion of progesterone from the corpus luteum of the ovary is intermittent, and can vary as much as 30 ng/ml. in 30 minutes. Also, low levels of progesterone are found in women who are not ovulating, although they do not necessarily suffer from premenstrual syndrome. However, a blood test to estimate the level of the binding capacity of the sex hormone binding globulin (SHBG) has proved valuable in premenstrual syndrome. My daughter, Dr Maureen Dalton, showed in 1981 that 50 women suffering from severe, well-diagnosed premenstrual syndrome all had SHBG binding levels below the normal 50–80 nmol/1DHT when compared with 50 healthy women who were adamant they did not suffer any premenstrual symptoms (Fig. 7).

Furthermore her work showed that SHBG levels rise when progesterone is administered, and the greater the dose of progesterone the higher the SHBG level (Fig. 8).

Later work showed that if progestogens were administered the SHBG levels were lowered. There are, however, limitations to the use of this test, for the woman whose blood is to be tested must be free from all medication (which includes analgesics, oral contraceptives, laxatives and vitamin preparations), must not be unduly obese or excessively hairy, and should not suffer from liver or thyroid disease. Furthermore the blood must be centrifuged and stored frozen until analysed by the purified two-tier method, which is at present only available at a few specialized centres in Britain.

Diagnostic Pointers

The menstrual chart must be completed for two or three months before a diagnosis of premenstrual syndrome can be made, and the SHBG test is not universally available. In selecting women for clinical trials into premenstrual syndrome, daily recording for two months is the minimum, but there are occasions when one is anxious to make a rough diagnosis earlier. This can be done by consideration of the characteristics of women with premenstrual syndrome, and are usually referred to as 'diagnostic pointers'.

Medical students are taught that the onset of the premenstrual syndrome is linked with PPPA – puberty, pregnancy and the pill, and after amenorrhoea or absence of menstruation, such as occurs after anorexia nervosa or after serious illnesses or accidents. In the young adolescent it may result in an unexpected change of personality. One mother wrote:

'For three weeks of the month our daughter is charming,

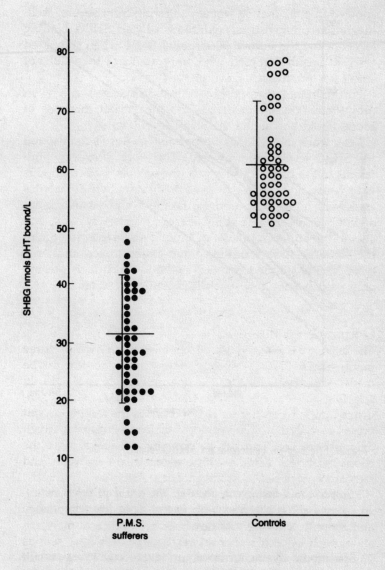

Fig. 7 SHBG-binding capacity in 50 patients with severe premenstrual syndrome compared with 50 controls

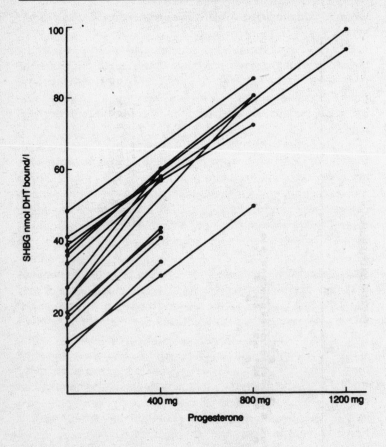

Fig. 8 Effect of progesterone on SHBG levels

capable and intelligent, then for the few days before her period she is sharp-tongued, impossible to live with and seems to be boiling with rage.'

Spasmodic dysmenorrhoea, or severe colicky spasms of pain which start with the onset of menstruation, is unusual in sufferers of premenstrual syndrome (see Chapter 8), and because menstruation is painless and a non-event many women initially fail to make the connection of their other symptoms with menstruation.

When, during pregnancy, menstruation stops and the blood level of progesterone rises some 30 to 50 times the peak level reached during the premenstruum, women with premenstrual syndrome lose their symptoms. Many a husband has exclaimed, 'I wish my wife could be forever pregnant.'

Premenstrual syndrome may start when the woman is on the pill, or during the week when she is off it, but complaints are likely to be more marked, and the bright and dull days more accentuated, when pill-taking ends. Then the woman resumes her normal menstrual cycle, which may well be three or five weeks and not the precise 28 days ordained by the makers of the pill. Marriage or the beginning of a relationship is often given as the time at which premenstrual syndrome started, but in these cases it may be that the observant partner has noticed mood swings and the other symptoms and related them to menstruation, when the woman had not noticed the connection earlier. Pill-taking may have coincided with the marriage. Some women claim that their premenstrual syndrome started only after they were sterilized, and many women insist that their premenstrual syndrome has increased in severity since sterilization. Radwanska, Hammond and Berger of Illinois University showed that after women had the simple operation to block their fallopian tubes they subsequently produced less progesterone from their ovaries.

Age and pregnancy are two factors which tend to make the symptoms of premenstrual syndrome become worse and last longer, so it may be first diagnosed in the thirties. In fact in 1963 Dr T S Lloyd suggested the name 'Mid-thirty Syndrome' for this same collection of symptoms related to menstruation, but this title would be unfair to those who also suffer during adolescence and their twenties. This increase in severity is more marked in the years just before the menopause, so much so that all too often the premenstrual mood swings are blamed on the menopause; a woman of fifty years exclaimed, 'I've been in the menopause for the last fifteen years; when will it ever end?' It is more likely that she has been suffering from undiagnosed premenstrual syndrome for the last fifteen years.

During adult life sufferers tend to have large weight swings exceeding 28 lb., although swings of 50 lb. or more are not unusual. The lowest ever weight since leaving school is subtracted from the highest ever, non-pregnant weight. It is irrelevant whether at the time of interview the individual is obese or slim.

Sufferers have difficulty in going long intervals without food, especially in the premenstruum, and may notice that this is when they become faint, excessively tired, panicky or irritable. They also tend to suffer from uncontrollable premenstrual food cravings and binges, especially when they have deliberately refrained from food for a long time or when weight reducing. This tendency is not due to a personality failure but the result of the hormonal factor. It even occurs in baboons in the jungle. They go up into the trees and, in isolation, gorge unlimited amounts of honey during their premenstruum.

The tolerance to alcohol in premenstrual syndrome sufferers also varies during the cycle. Sufferers usually find that a favourite alcoholic drink taken daily will cause intoxication only in the premenstruum.

If the woman gives many positive answers to the diagnostic pointers there is every likelihood that in two months she will return with a positive chart. There are occasions when it may be worth giving a patient a therapeutic trial with progesterone before waiting for a definitive diagnosis, but both the doctor and the patient should be aware that a positive diagnosis has not been made and, of course, the patient cannot be a candidate for any clinical trials.

An analysis was made of the final diagnosis in over 200 women who attended the premenstrual syndrome clinic. Its conclusions were that while the menstrual chart is the only reliable diagnostic method for premenstrual syndrome, it also demonstrated that the SHBG estimation was more specific, more sensitive and had a greater predictive value than the checklist score of diagnostic pointers.

Premenstrual Tension

Tension may be described in many ways, but the tension which occurs in the premenstrual syndrome has three parts to it: depression, tiredness and irritability. These three parts are always present in premenstrual tension although one of them may be more obvious than the others but only temporarily so. Dr Billig, in 1952, aptly described the depression as 'the world looks like a sour apple', the tiredness as a 'fall in energy' and the irritability as feeling 'crabby', and there are plenty of women who know exactly what he means.

These three symptoms may be interwoven, with each one of equal importance as DOROTHY's letter shows:

'Premenstrual tension has been present throughout my reproductive life. I have seen my doctor many times but he has really been unable to help. Perhaps predictably, the condition had grown steadily worse in the years just before the marriage break-up, and much, much worse since. The strain is very great and well nigh unbearable during the premenstrual time. I do not batter my children physically but I do verbally and I think that that can be almost as damaging, although I do try to explain to them why I behave as I do and apologize for it. The trouble begins as early as twelve to fourteen days after the beginning of the last period; the first sign is a disturbance of sleep. I get violent dreams and often wake and when it is time to get

up feel as though I have had no rest at all. The other half of the cycle I sleep perfectly soundly. Then I become so tense I positively shake and am so nervy and irritable that I am sorry for anyone who has to live with me. Quite often my head starts to pound for no obvious reason such as I have not been running or indulging in any violent exercise. I feel listless and apathetic and often fall asleep during the day; on the other hand the other half of the month I am energetic, hard working and clear headed. The onset of the period releases the tension but triggers off headaches which fluctuate from day to day for a couple of days. I cry at the drop of a hat during all this period and find it hard to deal with any of the many problems objectively. Although I have been very depressed, I have never been put out of action, thanks probably to the good professional help. Apart from this misery I am healthy and active and very rarely ill.'

Premenstrual tension, popularly abbreviated as PMT, is only one aspect of premenstrual syndrome, which includes the bodily, physical or somatic symptoms as well as the psychological ones.

Some try to cope with it alone; a competent boutique manager wrote:

'For many years I have managed to keep my PMS a secret, but increasingly I have found it more difficult to suppress. Friends have commented on unexpected changes in behaviour and total irrational responses to situations. I feel desperate and helpless that I am no longer able to manage my PMS, but it appears to be a dominant factor in my life today. Normally I am quite a positive and optimistic person, and they call me "Bubbles".'

The tension may come on quite suddenly with an inability to relax and generally feeling uptight. One housewife complained that when she was in this state she seemed to tremble so much that she even had difficulty in threading a needle. Frequently women are shy of mentioning premenstrual tension to their doctor, thinking that it is a common and minor complaint. Instead they present what is known by the medical profession as a 'passport symptom', or a somatic symptom like a headache or backache or 'flu, which they consider is more acceptable to the doctor. One mother wrote:

> 'When I go to the doctor I am always conscious that I am not physically ill and so perhaps do not want to tell him all my, to other people, petty feelings. After all, one does not want to admit being a failure as a wife and mother.'

Sometimes the tension reaches almost manic proportions with agitation and restless energy so that the woman cannot ease down, she keeps walking up and down, or won't stop talking and just repeats herself endlessly.

One husband was upset because:

> 'It's no use trying to tell her to relax, she just keeps repeating herself and won't stop talking. New thoughts keep tumbling out. She accuses me of all sorts of things. She just goes on and on and on.

Premenstrual tension, like all other symptoms of premenstrual syndrome, is always worse at times of stress. None of us can totally free ourselves from the stresses of daily life, such as those occasioned when extra work is demanded of us, or when something occurs which hampers our normal activities, or when friends or relations are involved in some misfortune or accident. The usual reaction to any of these stresses will be to cause an increase in the premenstrual tension when the time of the next menstruation approaches. On the other hand good news will tend to ease the tension, and a winning bet or lottery ticket can be most beneficial in relieving premenstrual tension, but only for a month or two.

Depression

The depression may be so mild that the actual word is not used or is even denied. However, the woman may admit to feeling fed up, down in the dumps, that she can't laugh easily and has difficulty in smiling, or that the whole world is against her and nobody cares. On the other hand, premenstrual depression may range to the other extreme, with a black cloud of depression interfering with concentration so that even the simplest of tasks, like reading or playing board games, become impossible, and with the ever-present possibility of suicide. This risk of suicide should always be fully appreciated.

One husband wrote describing his wife's depression: 'I feel her life is at risk, she dreads these times so much it colours her whole life. She feels there is no hope.' A mother described her 20-year-old daughter's depression:

> 'These occurrences are so regular that for years I have associated them with periods. But when she approaches her doctor, usually in a state of panic, she is either told to go away and pull her socks up, or is given tranquillizers and on at least three occasions she has taken the lot and has had to have her stomach pumped out. When she is in this state she often proves violent and smashes things or hits her boy-friend. She also swallows vast quantities of alcohol and then sometimes cuts her wrists, always in the wrong direction. When she is herself after a period she is such a nice, kind and good-natured person.'

An American secretary has ended her full description of premenstrual depression with the statement: 'The sad thing is that although suicide thoughts cross my mind at this time I am a very happy person ordinarily.'

The MacKinnons, a husband-and-wife team of doctors, showed as long ago as 1956 that successful suicides among women predominated during the premenstruum. Studies of attempted suicide undertaken in hospitals in London and Delhi and by Samaritans in Los Angeles have confirmed that half of all women's attempts at suicide are made during the four days immediately before or during the first four days of menstruation.

Although women make more attempts at suicide than men, the men succeed more frequently, but this masculine success rate gradually disappears after the age of 50 years. Dr John Pollitt, speaking at the Royal Society of Medicine in 1976, suggested the following:

> 'Perhaps one reason for the female's lack of success is that the majority of attempts are made during the premenstrual phase or menstruation. Killing oneself is not easy; success requires careful planning. Women in the premenstrual phase show a marked tendency to be careless, thoughtless, unpunctual, forgetful and absent-minded. This inefficiency at a time when they are more likely to try to end their lives may result in a disproportionate failure.'

Every suicidal gesture should be taken seriously, as just before and during menstruation a sufferer's mood may deteriorate so suddenly that an attempt may be made at a most unexpected moment. The attempt may end the life, even though it was only intended as a cry for help, or it may result in permanent damage even harder to cope with than the condition at the time of the attempt. Drug overdoses may result in permanent liver or kidney damage, and when a woman throws herself under a train or from a high window the scarred face and broken limbs are ever-present reminders of the event which made life so intolerable. One patient produced her diaries with a record of 40 overdose attempts; each one had needed hospital admission and had occurred during her premenstruum, those four fateful days before menstruation.

EDITH, a 24-year-old personal assistant, wrote:

> 'On December 6th, realizing how dangerous the premenstrual effects were, I felt in great need of help. Unfortunately my group meeting was during this time and did not

*help me at all. After the meeting I rushed home, hid from
my boy-friend whom I saw in the High Street, and intended
again to overdose. Fortunately two friends arrived on the
scene and by the time they left it was all over and I had
started to menstruate.'*

When women, and particularly young girls, are in the
depths of despair they may occasionally resort to self-muti-
lation with such acts as slashing their wrists, abdomen, neck
or face, or shaving their scalp or eyebrows. When they injure
themselves severely they apparently experience no pain and
appear to be anaesthetized during the process. Self-muti-
lation is rare in men, and although it can occur in any woman
it appears to be most frequent among young sufferers of
premenstrual syndrome, so much so that when self-muti-
lation occurs it is important to first eliminate the diagnosis
of premenstrual syndrome before resorting to routine anti-
depressant therapy.

Depression can be an emotion, such as when we hear of
the death of a near friend or other bad news, but it can also
be an illness when it affects all the bodily functions as well.
The symptoms of a depressive illness are similar in premenstrual depression, but there are differences, one being in the
timing. Whereas in a depressive illness the symptoms are
present day after day throughout the entire month and may
last for weeks, months or years, in premenstrual depression
the symptoms are measured in days and do not last longer
than 14 days, for after menstruation the woman is her
normal, happy, energetic self. Another important difference
is the marked irritability which accompanies the premenstrual depression. Premenstrual depression increases with
age after 26 years and is common among single women.

Depression is best thought of as a disease of 'loss' for there
are losses of happiness, interest and enthusiasm, of memory,
energy, sleep and sexual arousal. One feels a loss of security
and adequacy and a loss of the powers of concentration, so
that it becomes difficult to read a book or follow a television
programme. There is a loss of self-control, and an inability to

control one's tears, behaviour, appetite or decision-making. There is a loss of insight and an inability to realize, in the case of premenstrual depression, that very shortly the symptoms will pass during the course of menstruation and that there will be a return to normality.

Tiredness

'What worries me most is that I get so slow and stupid before my periods.' This comment by a journalist is echoed by many who find the lethargy, exhaustion and prostration so difficult to cope with during the premenstruum. The 'can't-be-bothered' attitude takes over and disrupts the programme for the day until in the end 'everything goes'.

FRANCES, a 32-year-old working mother, hated the tiredness most and wrote:

> 'The worst and most worrying symptom is the feeling of apathy which descends on me; all physical and mental activity becomes a real effort and all I want to do is curl up in a corner away from everyone and all my responsibilities. I find it quite frightening that I cannot think clearly or quickly and feel mentally dulled. These symptoms get increasingly worse and a couple of days before a period I feel quite ill. The first day of a period I feel a bit headachy and tired, but then it is like a weight being lifted off me and for two weeks or so I feel really fine.'

This tiredness may lead on to withdrawal and a wish to hide away in a corner, so aptly described by a secretary as: 'Total withdrawal from all social contacts and withdrawing into myself – despite living with friends I often find myself not wanting to speak unless absolutely necessary and often only managing one or two sentences.'

Again the tiredness may vary in severity from the typist who cannot remember what she is writing and fills her wastepaper basket with her typing errors to the executive who feels unable to compose letters and stares all day at a blank sheet of paper. A mother of two boys, aged one and three years old, wrote:

> 'When I am bad I stay in bed all day. One day last holiday I felt so bad I could not bear to lift my sons or get them dressed so the poor children had to stay in bed the whole day. I just cried and told them how sorry I was that I could not help them at all. I fear the little ones who have known me like this may grow up into disturbed children, but I promise you I'm quite normal at other times in my cycle.'

One woman, as yet unknown to me, asked for an appointment, and when describing her tiredness added:

> 'I seem to be in a daze on those days, can't do anything right – more than once I've crossed the road to go to the convenience and found myself in the Gents.'

Another housewife confessed that:

> 'Just before a period, for about ten days, a sleepiness takes over me and all I want to do is sit down and sleep, so therefore no housework or proper cooking gets done.'

It is the premenstrual tiredness which is responsible for the drop in mental ability before menstruation. At one boarding school it was possible to study 1,561 weekly grades of school-children and compare them with the previous week's grade. Each grade covered the marks of some seven to twelve different subjects. During the premenstrual week there was an average drop of 10% compared with a compensatory rise of 20% during the week immediately following menstruation, as shown in Fig. 9 (page 44). This effect is also evident in examination results.

Irritability

It is those who are nearest to a sufferer of premenstrual irritability who suffer most from her short fuse and explosions over trivial matters, and this is usually not only the nearest but also the dearest, which means the husband, children or parents. As one wife said:

> 'Pity those around me when the least things upset me, I hate everyone, shouting and picking quarrels, and the whole world gets on my nerves and I can only look at it with a jaundiced eye.'

Premenstrual irritability is commoner in the married woman, and the husband naturally has problems trying to calm a supersensitive, edgy, irrational and agitated woman during these days of each cycle. Too many end up with visits to the marriage-guidance counsellor or in divorce.

The following three quotations taken from women's letters received suggest that the husband has obviously suffered as much as his wife:

> 'I have been suffering from premenstrual tension for some years now; recently it came to its height. In July I was in my usual depressed state and being angry I didn't know what to do with myself, I just lost my temper . . . I kicked the door and required forty stitches in my leg. My husband is at his wits' end not knowing what to do with me, not knowing what I'm going to do next, and is ready to leave me after being married only eighteen months. I keep telling him that I'll be good next time, but I never am and just can't control myself.'

> 'Last Saturday I deliberately smashed all the dishes after clearing the table. I started menstruating in the evening. My general practitioner puts it down to my Irish temper. I get so depressed, hateful, horrid, tired, I stay in bed, shout and I could go on and on like this. It is my husband who asked me to write for help.'

'At thirty-two there is very little hope for me except the change; I have a history of suicide attempts, child and husband bashing and many rows with a long-suffering doctor, who has been accused by me of many crimes at my worst, such as neglect, attempted manslaughter amongst them. I have taken many prescribed anti-depressants in massive doses.'

If one sees a patient shortly after an aggressive outburst, like those described in the last three letters, it is possible to get full details of the time at which food has been taken during the day. It is a common finding that the irritability is always worse when, in addition to the closeness of menstruation, there has been a long interval since the last meal, causing the blood sugar level to fall (see discussion on blood sugar levels, pages 154–6). When patients are asked at what time of day their irritability rockets, it is usually in the late morning if breakfast has been missed, or when preparing the evening meal or waiting for the husband's return if he is later than usual. Often the wife has only had a sandwich, or possibly just cheese and an apple, at midday and is then at her wits' end, having eaten nothing else in anticipation of an evening meal with her husband. These sudden explosive outbursts of irritability or aggression can usually be helped by ensuring that small meals are taken at intervals of three hours. In two recent cases of murder and one of infanticide it was noted that in each case no food had been taken for nine hours.

At the height of the tension there may be true confusion with memory loss, so that the woman is unaware of her actions or surroundings. Indeed she may bitterly refute any action, for she has no memory of it. The following notes made by a patient show how extreme the confusion may be and how it may well represent temporary insanity.

'From the 4th onwards severe depression with secretive confusion. On the 7th I planned to kill my mother and myself. I wrote suicide notes to all concerned and I took

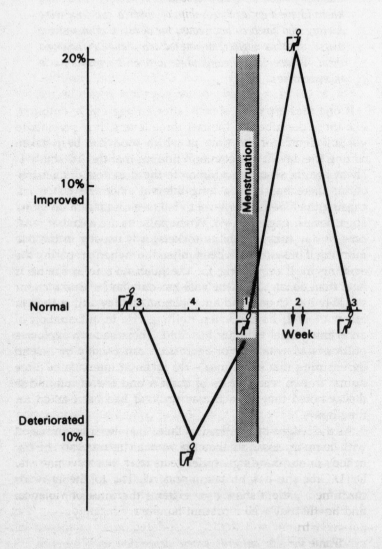

Fig. 9 Variation in schoolgirls' weekly grades with menstruation

certain prescribed drugs that I thought would work. I do not know whether I would have done it as my friend, with whom I have a good relationship, discovered that they were missing and flushed them down the toilet. It took quite a few days before I realized how bizarre the whole episode was. The loss of appetite, need for alcohol, aggression, lack of interest and swollen glands continued until menstruation started on the 9th. These notes are written on the 18th, when my mind is clear.'

It is not surprising that premenstrual tension with its irritability and confusion frequently leads to brushes with the law. There are those cases of assault where in a sudden fit of temper a woman throws a rolling-pin at her neighbour, a typewriter at her boss, or tries to bite off a policeman's ear. There are the cases of baby-battering, husband-hitting and homicide as seen in the examples already quoted. Becoming drunk and disorderly when under the influence of alcohol or drugs may also lead to the charge of assault. In France it is recognized that premenstrual tension may be so acute and so violent as to be classed as 'temporary insanity' in courts of law.

My British survey in 1961 of 156 newly committed women prisoners revealed that 49% had committed their crime during the paramenstruum, and in fact premenstrual syndrome was present in 63% of these women who committed their crime during the paramenstruum. Theft accounted for the highest proportion, with 56% of crimes being committed during the paramenstruum, while the alcoholics charged with being drunk and disorderly were a close second at 54%. In the same women's prison 20 years later, two psychiatrists, Dr D'Orban and Joy Dalton (no relation to the author), confirmed these statistics in relation to crimes of violence, finding that 44% had committed their offence during the paramenstruum and that 34% suffered from premenstrual syndrome.

The Parisian police noticed early this century that 84% of crimes of violence had been committed during the premenstruum or menstruation. This was confirmed by a similar study in New York which showed that 62% of crimes of violence occurred during the premenstruum.

Dr Morton and his colleagues working in Westfield State Prison in America showed that it was worthwhile treating the inmates of prison and reformatory if they suffered from the premenstrual syndrome. He found that treatment resulted in an increased work output, less punishment for disobeying rules and an increase in general morale. The question may well be asked, what benefit will a woman or society gain from a prison sentence or fine, if she is unable to control her premenstrual irritability or confusion? Unfortunately, if these premenstrual syndrome prisoners remain untreated they will usually serve their full sentences without remission for good conduct, since their symptoms get the better of them each premenstruum and cause further trouble whilst in prison.

5

Waterlogged

For some women, the days from ovulation to menstruation are characterized by bloatedness, heaviness and/or a gain in weight. The bloatedness is a sensation caused by the fluid outside the cells seeping into and expanding individual cells, so it does not necessarily mean that there is a gain in weight. The weight gain may be due to an accumulation of water in the tissues and cells of the body because only part of all the water that is taken in during that fortnight is passed out from the body; some remains and gradually accumulates. Not only is water retained but so may sodium, while potassium may be lost. It should be stressed that water retention is only one of the many symptoms of the premenstrual syndrome, and many women never experience it at all even though they may suffer from severe premenstrual syndrome.

The commonest sign of water being retained in the body is an increase in weight, which may average 4 to 7 lb. above the normal weight (Fig. 10), but of course it may well be more, even 10 to 12 lb. The normal weight is that which is taken during the postmenstruum and gains and losses of up to 3 lb. are usually considered within normal limits for women. Dr Thomas, of America, has documented a case of one woman who gained between 12 and 14 lb. each premenstruum and then lost it all together with an excessive output of 9 pints of urine on the first day of menstruation, the excessive urine output continuing for the next few days of

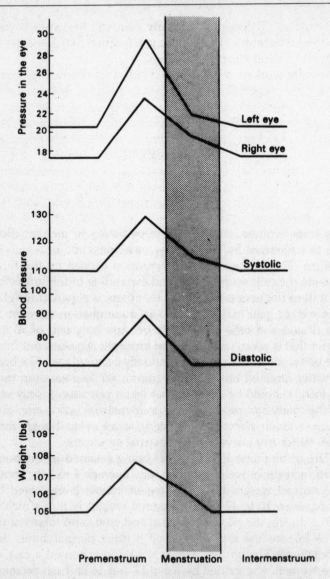

Fig. 10 Fluctuations during the menstrual cycle in weight, blood pressure and pressure in the eye of a sufferer of premenstrual syndrome

menstruation. Those who regularly gain and lose very large amounts of water irrespective of menstruation may be suffering from 'cyclical idiopathic oedema'.

The early workers on the premenstrual syndrome believed that the premenstrual weight-gain was an index of the severity of the premenstrual symptoms, but this is definitely not the case. In fact Dr Bruce and Professor Russell examined 34 women at Maudsley Hospital, London, who had complained of premenstrual symptoms, carefully measuring their weights, the amount of fluid they took in and the amount they passed out, and found no relationship. In fact they wrongly concluded that premenstrual syndrome was a purely psychological condition.

Apart from the gain in weight, the water retention shows itself in different tissues, with varying effects, as experienced by GLADYS who wrote:

'The pattern of a 5 lb. weight rise at period times makes me so bloated that it turns me out of my favourite slacks and makes me feel ready to burst. My breasts become enlarged and sore, needing a larger size bra, my eyes sink back and I get dark rings under the eyes. There is extreme fatigue, both physical, so that I can hardly put one foot before the other, and mental, so that I feel incapable of dealing with the children I teach. I am subject to quite black depressions caused by trivial things going wrong. I get throbbing and severe headaches in the week preceding the period and always during the first three days of bleeding. I do a full-time job, look after the home and three children, go to evening classes, I also paint and do flower arranging, so you can see I do try to fight it.'

Breast Soreness

Complaints of breast soreness with enlargement and tender nipples are common, and all too frequently this leads to fear that this may be a sign of cancer of the breast. It is definitely not related to cancer in any way. It is more that the breast tissue is getting ready in the hope that following ovulation a pregnancy will occur and the breasts will be needed for breast feeding. It must be emphasized that not all cases of breast tenderness are due to premenstrual syndrome. It only comes into this category if cyclical soreness is present in the premenstruum with complete absence of pain after menstruation. Breast engorgement present throughout the month but more marked in the paramenstruum may be caused by an increased output from the pituitary of the hormone prolactin. It is possible to measure the blood prolactin level and, if this is raised, treatment with bromocriptine may be beneficial. It must not be forgotten that the breasts are sexually charged areas and when the woman is having problems in her sex life her breasts may become more sensitive. Nipple sensitivity, as opposed to breast tenderness, may result from taking vitamin B6, even low dosages over a long period (see page 220).

Fluid Retention

The extra water in the tissues can cause the ankles and the fingers to swell so that shoes have to be discarded and rings removed. There may be swelling of the gums so that dentures no longer fit. The skin coarsens and becomes blotchy, contact lenses won't fit and hair becomes lank. One model who refused to accept work during the premenstruum said: 'I look my very worst, my skin won't take make-up, my face goes stiff and I can't move gracefully with those extra pounds of weight!'

The exact place where the water accumulates varies in different women and at different times in their life. The most severe symptoms result from water accumulating in a small unstretchable area, such as when water accumulates in the labyrinth of the inner ear and causes giddiness, when it enters the eyeball causing a raised pressure inside the eye and severe pain, and when it occurs inside the unyielding bony skull causing headaches. The sinuses are air spaces within the bones of the face. Air enters through the small entrance which is lined with cells of the mucous membrane, and when these are engorged and swollen the entrance to the sinus is blocked causing stale air to accumulate in the sinus, resulting in sinus headaches or 'vacuum headaches'. Water can also accumulate in the discs between the vertebrae of the spine, causing backache.

Sometimes there is a widespread distribution of the extra water which produces vague symptoms in the muscles, joints and soft tissues, causing generalized rheumatic pains, abdominal bloating and heaviness. The water is always in the cells or in the fluid between the cells. It is never free, although one patient imagined she could hear the water 'splashing within her abdomen', and another described how the abdomen was 'gurgling and swimming in water'. When the extra water accumulates in the fat and subcutaneous tissues there can be an appreciable gain in weight without any other complaints. This is most likely to happen in obese women.

One speaker, with his tongue in his cheek, observed at a medical lecture that, 'Today no woman suffers from obesity, only from water retention.'

Locating the Water

The actual site where the cells become swollen may vary from time to time depending on such factors as (1) anatomical abnormality, (2) heredity, (3) injury, and (4) infection. Thus a premenstrual sinus headache is more likely to occur in a woman whose cartilage in her nose is bent. Water is readily attracted to cells which have recently been injured or infected, so that after a fracture of the leg or arm it is usual to notice premenstrual swelling there for some months afterwards. If someone has recently had pneumonia it is likely that, if water retention occurs during the premenstruum, this may cause a return of the cough or breathlessness.

This water retention is often blamed for the depression and other symptoms which accompany it. HELEN, a 27-year-old unmarried accountant, wrote:

> *'I start to get tender, swollen breasts, usually 14 days
> (ovulation?) before the beginning of menstruation and I
> gain several pounds in weight. This makes me depressed
> and bad-tempered and when you feel like that you can't
> help getting annoyed with everyone around you.'*

Many of the symptoms of water retention are characteristically worse in the early morning, often waking the patient
from her sleep. This is especially so with migraine and with
the acute pain in the eyeball, mimicking glaucoma; and
asthma where there is swelling of the lining cells of the small
tubes of the lung. Some people are awakened by a feeling of
pins and needles, and perhaps numbness of their fingers.
This is because the nerve passes from the arm through a
narrow bony tunnel at the wrist, and when the surrounding
cells are swollen and waterlogged this nerve becomes con-
stricted. It is this which causes the odd sensations in the
fingers, and it is called 'a carpel tunnel syndrome'.

Nowadays, when we have many drugs which help to
increase the amount of urine passed, these would seem to
be a simple answer to the problem of water retention. Unfortunately the problem is not quite so simple. Although these
drugs (diuretics) can get rid of water, extra water forms again
quickly. It is rather like baling water from a boat with a hole
in it; it is better to bung up the hole and prevent further
water entering than merely to keep baling. Just as the balers
get tired, so do the water tablets. So the temptation, then, is
to use stronger and ever stronger drugs to get rid of more
and more water. But as mentioned at the beginning of the
chapter, the problem is not only that water accumulates but
also that potassium may be lost. Diuretics cause water and
more potassium to pass away in the urine so unless sufficient
potassium is added one may cause a marked lowering of the
blood potassium level resulting in an increase in the tiredness
and possibly also weakness of the legs. Doctors can do an
estimation of blood potassium level to know how much potassium is circulating in the blood at a given moment, but this
does not tell you how much potassium is present in the cells

or in the fluid between the cells, which is really what matters. There is now a new class of potassium-sparing diuretics which do not upset the potassium level, so these are the first choice if diuretics are really needed in premenstrual syndrome.

Another problem is that water retention does not cause premenstrual tension, depression, tiredness or irritability, so none of these symptoms will be relieved by diuretics. Actually diuretics are useful only in the short term until progesterone treatment can be given, or in the mild case where it is used sparingly with the addition of extra potassium if blood tests show low levels of potassium.

One often meets patients who have received diuretics continuously for many years and have become dehydrated. If diuretics are then stopped suddenly the patients complain bitterly of feeling bloated within a day or two of stopping. These patients need to be persuaded to tail off their diuretics gradually, by using them every other day, starting immediately after menstruation. After a month or two it may be possible to decrease the dose to every third or fourth day until it is only used when the weight-gain is really marked.

When a woman starts to gain weight there is the very natural temptation to start dieting. If her weight is above the ideal weight for her age and height this is all to the good, but she needs to be careful which diet she chooses. Not for her a diet of fruit juice and liquids only, as this will merely increase the fluid retention. If she tries to solve the problem by missing out meals, she risks the possibility that her blood sugar level will drop abnormally low, thus increasing the depression and irritability. Furthermore Dr Conn of America, who probably knows more than anyone about water, salt and potassium balance, has suggested that the body's reaction to a low blood sugar level is related to the amount of potassium in the cells. He has shown that the blood sugar level can be improved by correcting the potassium deficiency which may be present.

6

Monthly Headache

Many women like to jump on the bandwagon and claim that their own particular variety of headache only comes at period time. Undoubtedly menstruation is the most frequent time for migraine attacks in women, as seen in Fig. 11 in which the times of 935 migraine attacks are shown in relation to the days of the menstrual cycle. On the other hand those who can produce a three-month record showing a regular and definite relationship of the headache to menstruation have a much better chance of obtaining relief from progesterone treatment. In Fig. 12 it will be seen that Isobel's headaches last between seven and ten days before each period and are preceded by symptoms of tension, which eases off during the menstruation. Joan gives a different picture: her headaches only last one or two days, and there is no premenstrual tension, but the headaches all tend to come around the time of menstruation. Kathleen seems to have headaches every ten or twelve days; occasionally they do coincide with menstruation, but often they just come at any time. It is unlikely that Kathleen will benefit from hormonal treatment.

Characteristically, monthly headaches, which are likely to benefit from treatment with specific hormones such as progesterone, are those showing a definite relationship to menstruation in a three-month record; and those headaches which started either at puberty, after a pregnancy or while on the pill. These women are likely to be free from headaches

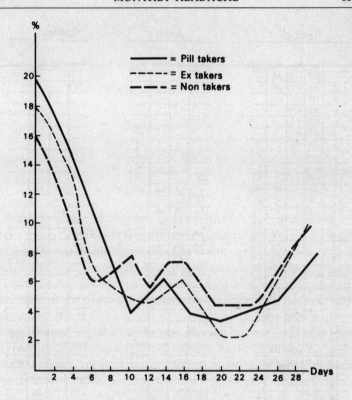

Fig. 11 935 migraine attacks in relation to the menstrual cycle

after the fourth month of pregnancy, and may well look back to the later months of pregnancy as the only time in their life when they knew what it was like to be free from headaches. But alas, these same women are also likely to say that immediately after the pregnancy the headaches returned worse than ever.

Women who find their headaches become worse while on the pill, or who have a tendency to headaches on the first or second day after stopping the course of pills, are likely to have menstrual headaches responsive to hormone treatment. The majority of these women with menstrually related head-

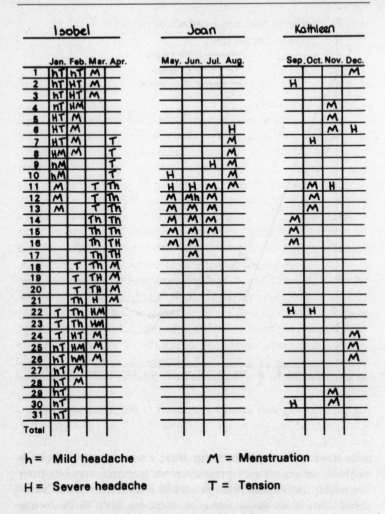

Fig. 12 Headaches in relation to menstruation

ache are also likely to find that after the menopause most of their problems come to an end.

The three common types of headaches related to menstruation are:

- 1 sinus or vacuum headaches
- 2 tension headaches
- 3 migraine

Vacuum Headaches

It is better to speak of 'vacuum headaches' rather than 'sinus headaches' as the latter are likely to be confused with the headache resulting from true sinusitis, which is due to infected material getting lodged in the sinuses. On the other hand the vacuum headaches are due to swelling of the cells at the entrance to the sinus, blocking the entry so that the stale air accumulates inside. These women may know that a headache is on the way when their nasal passages become blocked and it is difficult to breathe through one of their nostrils. There is tenderness or pressure over the sinuses, which are situated in the cheek bone and over the eyes (Fig. 13). The pain that results is made worse by bending down, and may last from one to seven days. In addition there may well be other signs of waterlogging such as gain in weight, bloated abdomen, shortness of breath or swollen ankles or fingers. These women would be wise to restrict their fluid intake to four cups of liquid daily and may benefit from nasal decongestants.

Tension Headaches

The tension headaches usually have a slow onset, so that the woman who is trying to chart it for the record may be uncertain whether the pain in the head is bad enough to call a headache. It usually starts after the beginning of the symptoms of premenstrual tension, irritability, tiredness or depression and eases off gradually during the course of menstruation. The pain from tension headaches has been described as 'like a steel cap pressing on my head' or 'like a heavy weight on top of my head' (Fig. 13). These women will find that the usual analgesics, such as aspirin or paracetamol, will only give ease for about four hours and then the

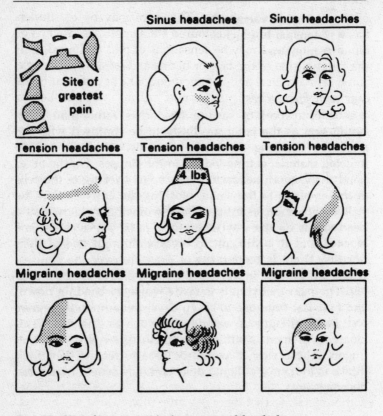

Fig. 13 Site of greatest pain in menstrual headaches

headache returns again, and the analgesic must be repeated. Treatment with progesterone (see Chapter 21) is the most valuable for this type of headache, and it also relieves the other symptoms of the premenstrual syndrome.

Migraine

Doctors like to divide migraine into two varieties, the classical and the common type. In the *classical* variety the patient has a warning or 'aura' lasting about twenty minutes before the onset of a severe headache. This aura may be of sudden flashes of lights, brightly coloured stars or stripes, a patch of blindness, or there may be sensations of pins and needles in the tongue, side of the face or hands and legs. Many people suffer both classical and common migraine at different times over the years. *Common* migraine has no aura and begins gradually, increasing in severity. The migraine may be accompanied by nausea or vomiting and extreme prostration and is likely to last between 24 and 48 hours, although some unlucky women find it lasts even longer.

Most migraine sufferers have a family history with a parent, brothers or sisters and uncles or aunts also suffering, so they do start with a predisposition to migraine. Nevertheless there are those among them whose attacks are related to menstruation and can benefit from simple advice and possibly also progesterone treatment.

In order to help women who have frequent or severe migraine attacks it is helpful to have full details of all they have been doing, and the times at which all foods have been consumed. (In practice an attack form, like that shown in Fig. 14, proves valuable and helps to isolate an individual trigger factor.) The trigger factor is the last straw which decides exactly when a migraine is going to occur in a susceptible woman. It is often the result of either going too long without food, so that there is a drop in the blood sugar level, or eating certain foods to which the sufferer is sensitive.

Too Long Without Food

When women are asked what sort of things start a migraine attack they often mention travel, theatregoing, and the day after a great event, such as when they have been working hard for several days preparing for a jumble sale, a wedding or special party. When the attack forms have been carefully filled in it is usually easy to spot if the migraine has been caused by too long an interval without food. Generally speaking five hours between meals is long enough for most women leading a normal energetic life, but women with

Name ....

Day of cycle ....

Date ....
Day of week ....
Time of onset ....
Duration ....
Days before next menstruation ....

During the 24 hours *before* an attack:–

(1) Did you have any special worry, overwork or shock?
(2) What had you done during the day?
      Normal work?
      Unusual activity?
      Extra tired?
(3) What food had you eaten and when?

Breakfast ....   Time ....
....
Mid-morning ....   Time ....
....
Lunch ....   Time ....
....
Mid-afternoon ....   Time ....
....
Supper ....   Time ....
....
Evening ....   Time ....
....
Bedtime ....   Time ....
....

Fig. 14 An attack form useful for isolating trigger factors in migraine

premenstrual syndrome will find that over three hours is too long an interval without food (see page 196). An overnight interval exceeding thirteen hours is usually considered the limit. After this length of time susceptible women, probably those already born with the tendency to migraine, will find they develop a headache. This explains why travel often causes a headache, for with frequent delays and long distances travelled, eating is often left for longer than usual. Similarly if one is busy with preparations for special events the food may all too easily be forgotten. And if you are giving the party, how easy it is to ensure that your guests have plenty to eat, but forget to take any food yourself.

Furthermore, one must consider not only the interval between meals but the amount of energy exerted during the interval, as the more energy is exerted, the quicker the blood sugar level falls. Overnight fasting is often the cause of a migraine attack on waking, and there are those migraine sufferers who say they cannot sleep long on holidays or at the weekend because they only wake up with a headache. Migraine is likely to occur when the evening meal is followed by some energetic sport or a brisk walk and no further food is taken before retiring to bed.

An example of this was noted in a receptionist, who was also a keen skater, and she normally had her evening meal at 6.30 p.m. On Thursdays she would be off to the rink for three hours of energetic enjoyment before retiring, but had no food after the evening meal. Every four or five weeks she would wake with a migraine on Friday mornings. The attacks occurred during the paramenstruum, but were triggered off by the long interval without food and the energetic skating.

Full information about the effect of a drop in blood sugar level is given on pages 154–6. If the attack forms suggest that the woman has had too long an interval without food, or has been too energetic for the amount of food she has had, it would suggest that the sudden drop in blood sugar may have triggered the attack. The question of treatment then becomes obvious: avoid fasting, remember to have an extra biscuit with the elevenses cup of coffee and with afternoon tea. Remember, too, that proteins, such as meat, fish and eggs, will keep the blood sugar up longer, while glucose sweets only cause a short, sharp rise in blood sugar level followed by a quick drop in level, and provide only a temporary benefit.

Foods Causing Migraine

Other women whose migraine attacks are not due to fasting, may find that they are sensitive to certain foods, the commonest of which are cheese, chocolate, alcohol and citrus fruits, but a few are sensitive to ripe bananas, pork, onions, fish and gluten. In these cases the migraine attacks do not occur immediately after the specific food has been eaten, but some 12 to 36 hours later. This is because the attack occurs not when the food is digested in the stomach, but rather when it is later broken down in the liver. In the liver these end products are finally broken down by the action of special chemicals known as enzymes and it would seem that if one particular enzyme is not present, then a wrong chemical action occurs, releasing substances capable of opening wide the blood vessels of the brain. These substances are known as vaso-dilating amines; two common ones are tyramine, which is present in cheese, and phenylethylamine, which is present in alcohol and chocolate, but there are also many other vaso-dilating amines, which can form from the wrong breakdown of everyday foods.

During the paramenstruum it seems that some women's sensitivity to vaso-dilating amines may be increased, so that although after menstruation they are able to take small amounts of the offending food, as menstruation approaches, or during menstruation, even a minute amount is sufficient to provoke an attack.

Women who come into this category would be wise if they tried to avoid the foods to which they are sensitive, remembering always that it is an individual problem. Foods which cause attacks in one individual will not necessarily cause attacks in another migraine sufferer. However, as mentioned earlier, there are often other members of the family who also suffer from migraine, so it is well worthwhile having a 'gathering of the clan' at which all blood relations who suffer from migraine can swop their ideas on the foods which they feel are detrimental to them. Often a common food can be discovered to which all members are sensitive.

Those who are sensitive to cheese will be happy to learn

that tyramine is not present in cream or cottage cheese, but only develops on maturing, so among the particular cheeses to be avoided are Stilton, Cheddar, Parmesan and processed cheeses. However, they should be aware that mature cheese is often hidden in quiches, mornay sauce and Italian dishes.

Red wine, sherry, port and champagne are probably the worst alcohols for causing migraine, while often it is possible to take a single glass of white wine with food without any after-effects. It is also worth considering the difference between grape and grain alcohols, for more people are sensitive to grape alcohols than to the grain alcohols like beer, vodka and whisky.

Chocolate is often added to rich fruit cakes or ginger cakes to give a good colour, and to coffee dishes to increase the flavour, so those who are sensitive to chocolate should be on their guard. Plain dark chocolate is more likely to provoke an attack than milk chocolate. How easy it is for those sensitive to citrus fruits to forget that this also includes mandarins and tangerines.

7

Recurrent Problems

My interest in premenstrual syndrome was first aroused within a few days of qualifying as a doctor in 1948, and whilst working as a locum to a general practitioner. In the early hours of the morning I received a call from a 34-year-old mother of three children, who had an acute attack of asthma. The husband, who opened the door, was most apologetic for calling the doctor out at such an hour, but added, 'Unfortunately it happens every month except when she's pregnant.' The woman certainly had a severe asthmatic attack and was quickly given an injection to ease her breathing. Driving home, the husband's words recalled my own migraine which also occurred once a month, just before menstruation, and my only time of freedom had been during my pregnancies. Later that day, a visit to the patient revealed that her first attack of asthma had occurred at the age of 17 years, coinciding with her first period, and she had an attack of asthma with each menstruation. The medical textbooks did not mention this possibility, but Dr Raymond Greene, who had helped me with my migraine, suggested that this patient should also be treated with progesterone. In those days only a doctor could give the injections, and during that first month, while giving the asthma patient her daily injections, I came across another woman with premenstrual asthma, two with premenstrual epilepsy and one with premenstrual migraine. So did the story of premenstrual syndrome begin.

In the early years it was essentially the bodily ailments which were noticed, with less appreciation of tension and other psychological symptoms. A survey in 1982 of 1,095 women being treated with progesterone for premenstrual syndrome, compared with the symptoms reported in the first article on premenstrual syndrome in the *British Medical Journal* in 1953, emphasizes the differences:

Year of survey	1953	1982
Percentage with symptom	%	%
Headache	69	33
Depression	6	35
Vertigo	13	3
Skin lesions	13	3
Bloatedness	6	31
Asthma	5	1
Epilepsy	5	1
Breast tenderness	2	21

The only way to identify a chronic recurring symptom as being part of the premenstrual syndrome is to chart it carefully together with the dates of menstruation for at least three months. If this was done more frequently there would be many more women whose asthma, epilepsy, migraine and host of other complaints would be identified as menstrually related and would then be eligible for relief by progesterone therapy. At present the list of symptoms which can, in some individuals, be related to menstruation proves to be endless and certainly covers all the systems of the body, so that all specialists, no matter what their discipline, are likely to come across its effects. In fact many of the symptoms are among the commonest that the specialist is called upon to treat. For instance the neurologist sees most patients with headaches and epilepsy, the dermatologist sees many patients with acne and boils, the urologist sees cystitis and urethritis, and so on.

Women with bodily, or somatic, symptoms related to menstruation will have the usual characteristics of the premenstrual syndrome: they will have the onset at puberty, after pregnancy, the pill; they will be free from symptoms in later pregnancy, and symptoms will be eased after the menopause. There will be a high number whose symptoms start after a pregnancy complicated by pre-eclamptic toxaemia, postnatal depression or sterilization.

While it will never be possible to give a list of all the possible symptoms which on occasion may be included in premenstrual syndrome, the common ones will be discussed (Fig. 15).

The premenstrual *asthma* appears to be caused by water retention in the cells lining the smaller tubes of the lung which become swollen and prevent the free entry of air into the minute air sacs. Thus the cause is not necessarily allergic, and in fact these patients do not all respond to sodium cromoglycate (Intal) inhalers as do those whose asthma has a definite allergic basis. Premenstrual asthma is particularly common in women in their thirties and forties. Usually the women will volunteer that their attacks are brought on by stress and tension, but they may not yet have related it to premenstrual tension. In the special asthma clinics in hospitals it is usual to find that about one-third of women in childbearing years have menstrually related asthma. Two women, aged eighteen and forty-two, have been treated at the Premenstrual Syndrome Clinic, University College Hospital, London. They had both had over twenty admissions to intensive care units for acute asthma, until an alert ward sister noticed that the attack always occurred premenstrually. Both have since been free from asthma on progesterone treatment.

One of the most satisfying experiences is to be able to diagnose and treat a woman with premenstrual *epilepsy*. They can be treated with progesterone and freed from all anticonvulsant tablets with their many and unpleasant side

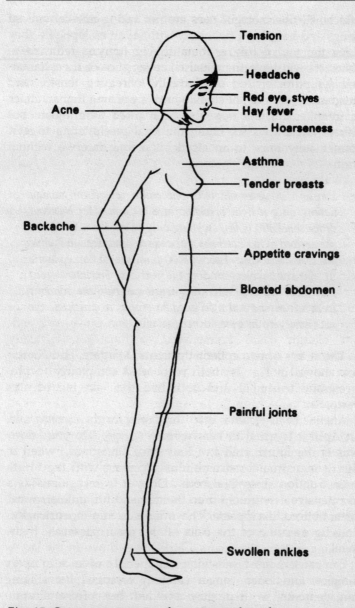

Fig. 15 Common symptoms of premenstrual syndrome

effects. Furthermore, if they are not taking anti-convulsant drugs and have been two years without an epileptic fit, they have the joy of having their driving licences returned to them. It seems that premenstrual epilepsy is often a culminating symptom on top of gradually increasing tension and headache, so these patients do have a warning that an attack is imminent. There may also be marked weight-gain, but this is not always so. Often the final precipitating trigger, immediately prior to an attack, is a long interval without food.

> LAURA, 28 years old with one child, set off on holiday having only a light breakfast at 8.00 a.m. Her husband drove some 300 miles, stopping only to ask the way. When she arrived at her hotel she had a nasty headache, and while she was unpacking at about 5.00 p.m. she had an epileptic fit. She started menstruating the next day. She later agreed that there had been mounting tension during the previous week which she had attributed to trying to finish all the necessary jobs in time for her holiday.

The charts of two epileptic patients, Margaret and Nancy, are shown in Fig. 16; both responded completely to progesterone treatment and both had their driving licences restored.

Rhinitis or *hay fever* is often mistaken for the *common cold*. In April it is usual to hear women saying, 'Do you know, this is the fourth cold I've had since Christmas,' when in fact it is a premenstrual rhinitis occurring with the fourth menstruation since Christmas. Once it is recognized as a premenstrual symptom then the demand for antihistamines or antibiotics disappears. The rhinitis is due to extra water causing swelling of the cells of the nasal passages. If the swelling of the cells occurs a little lower down in the larynx it can cause *hoarseness*, which is a special nuisance to opera singers. One opera singer carefully arranged her singing engagements so that they avoided her premenstruum. Another remarked that during the premenstruum the quality

Name MARGARET

#	Jan.	Feb.	Mar.	Apr.	May	Jun.
1		M				
2						
3	X					
4						
5	M					M
6	M					M
7	M				M	M
8	M				M	M
9	M				M	M
10					M	
11					M	
12					M	
13						
14						
15				M		
16				M		
17				M		
18				MX		
19			M	M		
20			M	M		
21		X	M	M		
22			M			
23		M	M			
24		M	M			
25		M				
26		M				
27		M				
28	M			*		
29	M					
30	MX					
31	M					
Total						

Margaret is 27 yrs old with 2 children, onset after 1st pregnancy

Name NANCY

#	Jan.	Feb.	Mar.	Apr.	May	Jun.	Jul.
1							
2							
3				X			
4					X		
5					M		
6			MX	M			
7			M	MX			
8			M	M			
9			X	MX	M		
10							
11		X					
12		M					
13	M	MX					
14	M	M					M
15	M	M					M
16	M	M			M	M	
17	M	M			M	M	
18	M	MX			M		
19	M	M			M		
20	M				M		
21					M		
22							
23							
24							
25							
26							
27							
28							
29					*		
30							
31							
Total							

Nancy is 28 yrs old, onset at puberty

M = menstruation
X = epileptic attack
* = progesterone treatment started

Fig. 16 Charts of two patients with premenstrual epilepsy

of her voice changed and she was unable to reach the high notes. This was corrected by progesterone therapy.

The loss of a sense of smell is probably more common than generally appreciated and is presumably due to extra water accumulating in the cells responsible for the sense of smell. The manufacturer of a special brand of anti-perspirant/deodorant noticed that women tended to change their brand after three or four weeks' use, complaining that it had ceased to function effectively. Market research showed that the dissatisfaction of the women was due to a premenstrual increase in sweating and vaginal discharge and a diminishing perception of the reassuring perfume of the anti-perspirant/deodorant product. This had led women falsely to believe that the product had lost its efficiency.

Giddiness or *vertigo* is a common complaint. In some surveys it occurred in a third of all sufferers of the premenstrual syndrome. It is most frequent among those who have had children and are approaching the menopause. The giddiness gets worse if she stoops and it may accompany a headache. The probable cause is excess fluid in the labyrinth of the ear, which is responsible for balance.

Similarly *fainting* is common just before menstruation, and is most likely to occur when there has been a long interval without food, or prolonged standing. It is common among teenage schoolgirls, who have missed their breakfast, and have to stand for a long time at the early-morning assembly.

Cystitis and *urethritis* are common symptoms during the premenstruum and may be caused by the increase in vaginal discharge and generalized pelvic congestion.

Joint and *muscle pains* may come back each month just before menstruation, last only a few days and then disappear without treatment. There may also be stiffness on waking in the morning, although this disappears within the hour. The pain is likely to be due to localized swelling of the cells, or to the failure of muscle relaxation during the time of premenstrual tension. The presence of water retention in many of these symptoms led to the mistaken theory that premenstrual syndrome was due to water retention, which could therefore be corrected by diuretics (water tablets). The effect of such treatment has already been discussed (pages 52–3).

There are many factors responsible for the formation of *varicose veins*, including a family tendency. However, when they first begin to appear they may only be visible in the premenstruum; later they may be painful only at this time of the cycle.

Boils, *styes* and *acne* are all common skin lesions which frequently come back each cycle just before menstruation. *Acne* is perhaps a special case. It is caused by the grease (or sebum) being too thick and too plentiful. This grease is produced by sebaceous glands in the skin and is excreted through the pores. If the grease is too thick it blocks the pores and causes acne. The skin only starts making grease, or sebum, at puberty, so in the first few years of its production there is often either too much or too little, or it is too thick or too thin. Gradually the body learns how to make the right amount. Oestrogen helps to slow down the production of grease, so acne often comes back at the time of falling oestrogen level, such as at ovulation and before menstruation. This also explains why acne usually improves · during pregnancy when there is plenty of oestrogen, and also in some women who are on the high-dosage oestrogen contraceptive pill.

Conjunctivitis, or red eye, may return each month due to causes other than infection. It is interesting that the association of conjunctivitis and menstruation was known as long ago as the sixteenth century.

Glaucoma is due to raised pressure within the eyeball. It can be caused by a narrowing of the opening through which the circulation fluid in the eyeball drains away, so it is not surprising to find that when there is water retention during the premenstruum there may be an excess accumulation of fluid within the eye and also difficulty in draining it away (Fig. 10). When this happens the pressure within the eye is raised, it becomes very painful and by pressure on the optic nerve may interfere with the sight. A survey of patients of menstruating age with closed angle glaucoma (where the drainage is blocked) at the Institute of Ophthalmology, London, revealed that 89% suffered from the premenstrual syndrome.

Uveitis and *iritis* are two other troublesome eye conditions which tend to flare up premenstrually and which respond so well to progesterone treatment.

Capricious appetite, food cravings and *binges* occurring at the height of premenstrual tension and water retention are well recognized. However great the self-control may be during the rest of the month, there come those days when she is 'overtaken by a demon and eats enough for a week in just one meal' or 'eats like a pig, stuffing on sweets'.

OLIVE wrote from America:

> *'My life swings between cycles of feasting and fasting. Having lived on a careful diet of only 750 calories for two weeks and lost 4lb. I had an uncontrollable urge, which got me out of bed, raided Mother's pantry and ate two loaves of bread with peanut butter, a packet of ginger biscuits and an apple tart.'*

Drs Smith and Sauder from McMaster University, Canada, studied three hundred nurses and confirmed the craving for food and sweets and the desire to eat compulsively during the times of premenstrual depression.

The actual foods chosen when there is a compulsive eating session are invariably carbohydrates and sweets, suggesting that the body's natural defence is coming into action to prevent a too severe or prolonged drop in blood sugar level (see pages 154–6).

Alcoholic bouts may be a feature of the paramenstruum. A survey of American female alcoholics revealed that 67% related it to the menstrual cycle and were able to abstain at other times; they all felt that their drinking habits had either started or increased during the premenstruum. During the paramenstruum the process of breaking down the alcohol appears to be slowed so that more accumulates in the bloodstream. Many women find they cannot hold their normal amount of alcohol at this time, which is unfortunate as it implies that care is needed when taking alcohol as a pick-me-up to relieve the depression and tension. Alcohol also helps sleep, but should not be used for this purpose during the premenstruum.

Dentists recognize that *ulcers in the mouth* commonly recur during the premenstruum, and these are sometimes accompanied by *ulcers in the vulva, vagina and anus*. Most opticians have learned that when making appointments for fitting *contact lenses* they must consider the time of the client's cycle, for fitting may prove troublesome during the premenstruum. Similarly hairdressers know that if a permanent wave hasn't taken, the chances are that it was done on the wrong day of the month.

Drug reactions are often reported during the premenstruum, and it always proves difficult to know exactly if it was due to the drug or a symptom of the premenstruum. When doctors are doing blind controlled trials of new drugs it can also produce confusion. Often one finds the dummy tablet effective, whereas the real drug causes headaches, increased drowsiness or nausea. But it may be because the dummy tablet is being taken during the postmenstrual week when the woman is feeling well, and the real tablet during the premenstruum and she is just reporting her normal premenstrual symptoms.

Mention should also be made of pain known as the *Mittelschmerz*, or middle pain, which may occur at the time of ovulation. This is usually a mild cramping pain in the lower abdomen on one side or the other, usually alternating month by month. It is due to the release of the egg cell from the ovary and possibly to the contractions of the tubes as the egg cell makes its way down to the womb. The pain only lasts a few hours, and may be accompanied by a vaginal discharge or even slight bleeding. Young girls are apt to mistake it for acute appendicitis, and more than one teenager has arrived at my surgery complete with a packed case so that she could be sent straight off to hospital. In fact there is no vomiting, no distension of the abdomen and none of the usual signs of guarding and localization of pain which the doctors normally look for when they examine an abdomen. It is important to get these girls to record the time of abdominal pain as well as the dates of menstruation so that they themselves can appreciate the relationship. Although ovulation occurs alternately on the right or left side, it is not completely regular. For instance, it may be right, right, left, right, left, left . . . so that at the end of the year it will probably have occurred an equal number of times on both sides. This pain, or sensation, should be regarded as Nature's signal that ovulation is occurring and indicating a favourable time for intercourse in those seeking to conceive, or a time for abstinence in those wishing to avoid a pregnancy.

8

Pain and Periods

A very welcome and much needed breeze of common sense wafted through the medical field when Drs Jean and John Lennane, a husband-and-wife team, pointed out in a well-reasoned paper on a group of disorders, which included period pain, that there is no justification for the old idea that 'it is all in the mind' and that there is no real scientific evidence for such a claim. Indeed, all the scientific evidence that existed pointed to a hormonal imbalance. They use a number of quotations from current medical textbooks which they suggest have led to an irrational and ineffective approach to the treatment of such disorders. These quotations include the following:

> 'It is generally acknowledged that this condition is much more frequent in the "highly-strung", nervous or neurotic female than in her more stable sister.'

> 'Faulty outlook . . . leading to an exaggeration of minor discomfort . . . may even be an excuse for not doing something that is disliked.'

> 'The pain is always secondary to an emotional problem.'

> 'Very little can be done for the patient who prefers to use

menstrual symptoms as a monthly refuge from responsibility and effort.'

The idea that period pains, or dysmenorrhoea, are purely psychological was put forward because there were no abnormalities to be detected on full physical or gynaecological examination, nor are there any suitable tests of hormone levels which can distinguish those who suffer once a month. However, gradually it is being realized that dysmenorrhoea is due to an imbalance of hormones.

There are two quite different, and indeed opposite, types of dysmenorrhoea, which are rarely differentiated by the general public, but it is essential to distinguish between them as the treatment of the two types is different. There is *spasmodic dysmenorrhoea*, which is characterized by spasms of abdominal pain, and *congestive dysmenorrhoea*, in which there is congestion of water or rather water retention. This latter type has all the characteristics of the premenstrual syndrome with the addition of period pains.

Spasmodic Dysmenorrhoea

When menstruation first starts at puberty no ovulation occurs nor is there any period pain. However, about two years later ovulation commences and then spasmodic dysmenorrhoea also begins in some women. Often, at the beginning, ovulation does not occur every month, but possibly only on alternate months, so period pains will only occur on alternate months. Spasmodic dysmenorrhoea is most frequent between the ages of 15 and 25 years. It ends abruptly after a full-term pregnancy, or it may gradually end with each period becoming less painful during the early twenties. The girl usually feels very well during the premenstruum and then is suddenly doubled up with severe spasms of pain in the lower abdomen on the first day of menstruation. The pain is colicky in nature, coming about every twenty minutes and lasting about five minutes – in fact they are similar to true labour pains. The girl obtains most relief by lying down curled up around a hotwater bottle, while aspirins may help to take the edge off the pain, and gin is the old-fashioned remedy. The pain may be so severe that bed is the only refuge, and pain may continue throughout the night preventing sleep. A monthly absence from work becomes the rule. The pain is easier on the second day and has passed by the third or fourth day. The distribution of pain is in the 'jock strap' area as shown in Fig. 17; in fact it covers the area served by the uterine and ovarian nerves. The severity of the

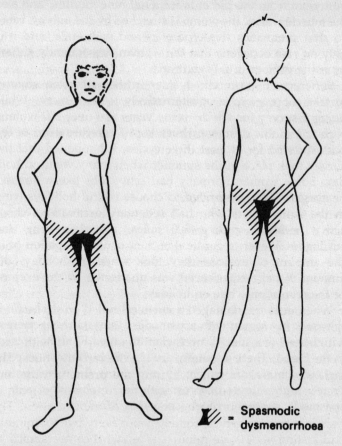

= Spasmodic
dysmenorrhoea

Fig. 17 Site of pain in spasmodic dysmenorrhoea

pain continues relentlessly month by month and is not
affected by stress. It may be helped, temporarily at least, by
an operation popularly known as a 'D & C', or a dilation and
curettage to stretch the opening of the womb. The girl is
often immature with sparse hair in her armpits and lower
abdomen, small breasts with pink nipples and acne.

It would seem that spasmodic dysmenorrhoea is due to
insufficient oestrogen for maturing and stretching the muscles of the womb. During pregnancy there is abundance of
oestrogen from the placenta for a full nine months, and also
the muscle wall of the womb is stretched by the unborn babe,
so after pregnancy this type of period pain ends, and it is
only on rare occasions that the woman subsequently suffers
from the premenstrual syndrome.

Sufferers of spasmodic dysmenorrhoea are often advised
to take more exercise or alternatively to relax more. While
doing a survey for *Which?* some years ago over 200 women
with spasmodic dysmenorrhoea kept a careful record of the
pain suffered for at least three cycles. It happened that the
survey took place in the summer when many went on holiday. Some women normally had active jobs like waitresses
or nurses, and they tended to choose restful holidays lying
in the sun. Others who had sedentary occupations chose
active holidays, cycling 500 miles, mountaineering and
surfing. However, regardless of their usual occupation or of
the amount of exercise they took while on holiday, the
amount of pain experienced was unaffected by the exercise
or the relaxation while on holiday.

When cells are damaged a chemical called *prostaglandin* is
released. In women with spasmodic dysmenorrhoea there is
a high level of a special prostaglandin called F2 alpha present
in the blood. There are many drugs available known as prostaglandin inhibitors which, by preventing the development
of too high a level of prostaglandin, inhibits the pain of
spasmodic dysmenorrhoea (see pages 202–3).

Congestive Dysmenorrhoea

Congestive dysmenorrhoea is the presence of heavy, continuous lower abdominal pain, during the last seven days of the premenstruum, which increases in severity on the first day of menstruation and then gradually eases, together with the end of the other premenstrual symptoms. The congestion was thought to be due to water retention. Congestive dysmenorrhoea is another presentation of the premenstrual syndrome. In contrast to spasmodic dysmenorrhoea, sufferers of the premenstrual syndrome may start with pain at their first menstruation and continue with it throughout their menstrual life, and the symptoms are present whether ovulation occurs or not. The pain is affected by stress, being worse when life in general is in turmoil and being eased by happy events. A 'D & C' brings no relief, nor does a pregnancy; in fact, the premenstrual symptoms may be worse after each pregnancy. Again in contrast to spasmodic dysmenorrhoea, the sufferers of the premenstrual syndrome are more mature and maternal, with large breasts and brown nipples. An interesting fact is that smoking tends to make this kind of pain worse.

Oestrogen administration increases the severity of the premenstrual syndrome, which responds to progesterone. Indeed excess progesterone administered to girls who have not borne children can cause spasmodic dysmenorrhoea. Thus, in theory, either type of dysmenorrhoea can be produced at will by overdosing with the wrong hormone, oestrogen or progesterone, which in itself proves that painful periods are not psychological but are due to hormonal imbalance.

While stressing the benefit which can be obtained from appropriate treatment of painful periods, the very exceptional woman, who does not ask for relief, should not be forgotten. A 19-year-old filing clerk, living in a slum dwelling in a suburb in East London, was visited on one occasion for 'flu. In conversation her mother mentioned that she also suffered from severe period pains each month and would be brought home from the West End in a taxi. My immediate response was that suffering of this calibre was no longer necessary today, whereupon the girl replied, 'Oh, don't! How else could I get a taxi ride once a month?'

Misplaced Cells

A rare cause of painful periods, which may come on with the first menstruation or after years of normal menstruation, and which affects only about one woman in twenty with dysmenorrhoea, is due to a condition known as *endometriosis*. The cells of the lining of the cavity of the womb, or endometrium, become displaced, and may either be found in the muscle wall or outer coat of the womb itself; in the ligaments around the womb; the ovary or tubes; the bladder or bowel; or anywhere in the lower abdomen. (Fig. 18 shows the relative position of the organs around the womb.) These endometrial cells lining the cavity of the womb have a unique ability to multiply, be shed, grow again and multiply in an endless cycle under the menstrual hormonal influence. Each time the lining cells are shed they pass out from the opening of the womb, into the vagina and out of the body as a menstrual flow. However, the misplaced cells are not able to be shed out of the body, and instead tend to accumulate as tiny cysts which later become inflamed and covered with scar tissue and adhesions. Each time thickening of the lining occurs during the premenstruum, these endometrial cells multiply, and as the cells are shed at menstruation more room has to be found within these cysts for the extra cells, so you can well understand that after a time it becomes a very painful condition with pain not only limited to the jock strap area, but all over the lower abdomen, possibly also affecting the bladder and rectum. In addition to the painful periods, endometriosis is characterized by extreme pain during thrusting at intercourse, which may diminish and stop all sexual desire, and also by infertility due to scar tissue forming around the ovaries and tubes. Doctors can diagnose the condition by the story of painful periods, pain at intercourse and infertility, and also by gynaecological examination

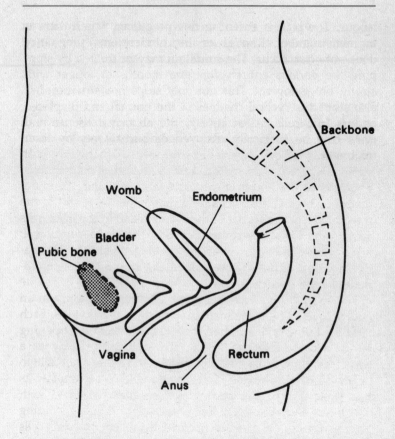

Fig. 18 The position of organs around the womb

and if necessary by laparoscopy, an operation in which a minute periscope is inserted through a small cut in the abdominal wall and the surgeon can then see for himself the tiny cysts and surrounding scar tissue.

Why the cells become displaced remains a mystery. It is possible that some were displaced during the developmental stage of the reproductive system in early foetal life, while it is also possible that some lining cells find their way through the fallopian tubes into the pelvis either at menstruation or labour. The pain is absent during pregnancy when there is no menstruation, although as already mentioned pregnancy does not often occur. The condition may be treated by stopping the periods entirely for nine months or longer with strong progestogens. This not only stops menstruation but also stops the cyclical changes in the normal and displaced endometrial cells. Alternatively, the abnormal tissues and cysts may be surgically removed or burnt away by laser treatment.

9

Awkward Adolescent

The menarche, or first menstruation, is an important milestone in any girl's life and demonstrates that she has an intact hormonal pathway from the hypothalamus and pituitary to the ovaries and womb. It is heralded over a period of some two years by the development of secondary sex characteristics such as breast development, skin and circulatory changes, the growth of pubic and armpit hair and changes of the body shape into the rounded female figure (Fig. 19). However, it is not the end of pubertal development, and only represents an approximately halfway stage.

The changes in the breast occur very slowly, from the first development of a small 'bud' under the nipple the size of a grape, and gradually increasing in size to full development. Often one breast develops slightly before the other, but although this discrepancy often causes so much worry that immediate medical advice is sought, there is no cause for alarm. In due course in the majority of cases both breasts will develop equally for the growth stimulus comes from hormones in the bloodstream.

In India and Sri Lanka the first menstruation is a cause for celebration as it represents the girl's attainment of full maturity and the beginning of her sexual and reproductive life. The occasion is marked by a change from wearing short dresses to dressing in colourful and beautiful saris. There are reports that in Pakistan the girls in some households were deliberately fed on a low-protein diet in order to delay the menarche, thus postponing the cost of a marriage which is expected to occur immediately the menarche has taken place.

The attitude taken towards this pubertal development depends very much on the culture of the society to which the girl belongs. In some societies, such as Japan and Hong Kong, where the subject is still very taboo, the girls obtain their information furtively from the pages of the popular press. On the other hand, in Britain today sex education is discussed so freely at home, at school and in the media, that when the menarche occurs it is almost a non-event. The only girl in a male-dominated family may be especially fearful of the menarche, which emphasizes the many differences between herself and her brothers and may increase the conflict over her developing femininity.

The age of the menarche is influenced by racial, genetic, dietetic, social and economic factors. In Britain the average

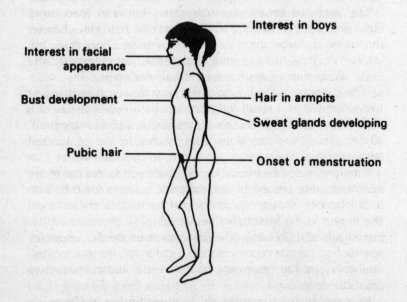

Fig. 19 Development at puberty

age of the menarche is 13.1 years, but it varies throughout the world, being highest in the Bundi tribe in New Guinea at 18.8 years and lowest in Cuba at 12.4 years. There is an early menarcheal age among British children attending special schools for the deaf and blind where menarche occurs at the average age of 12.2 years, and an even earlier menarcheal age among those with congenital abnormalities known to have started in early foetal life like spina bifida and rubella when the average age is 10.8 years. On the other hand the mentally disabled and those with Down's syndrome tend to have a later menarche. In Britain the range for normal children is from 10–16 years – in fact there is only one girl in a hundred who has not started menstruating by the age of 16 years. There has been a trend for the age of menarche to decrease since 1850 when it was 17.5 years, and this decrease is attributed to better nutrition. It is thought that the age of menarche has stabilized in the last twenty-five years.

The first menstruation usually lasts between three and eight days with an average of 5½ days, which is rather longer than most mothers expect it to be. There is then likely to be an interval of two or three months before the next menstruation. Only about four menstruations occur during the first year after the menarche, and gradually the cycle becomes shorter. Irregularity of periods is still quite frequent and at the age of 16 years, 20% of girls still have cycles which last longer than 40 days, and 33% have a prolonged bleeding lasting at least seven days.

Irregularities of menstruation are quite normal for the teenager and there are many quite normal reasons for this, but it can be very worrying for the girl herself. In these years she is not only adjusting to her developing feminine figure but she is also becoming more conscious of the opposite sex; as boy-friends come into the picture she becomes more interested in her own appearance, and these are often emotion-laden days.

In a single girl the cycle tends to be longer, perhaps 35 days, but as she begins to be stimulated by contact with boy-friends her cycle may shorten by a few days and reach nearer to the conventional norm, for the menstrual hormones are stimulated by male company. However, if she is then jilted and returns to female companionship her cycle usually returns to its original pattern.

One 19-year-old enquired:

> 'My periods were always very irregular with sometimes even eight weeks apart. When I first met John they became better and once as short as 28 days. Then we had an awful quarrel and I broke up with him. Since then my cycles only seem to come when they want to, every five or six weeks. Does it matter?'

At nineteen it does not matter, and probably even before she received a reply she would have found another boy-friend and menstruation would have become more regular again.

About two years after the menarche, ovulation occurs, not necessarily every month initially, but every two or three months, and gradually the cycles become more regular. It is with the onset of ovulation that spasmodic dysmenorrhoea can occur. This usually comes as a surprise to both the girl and her mother, as previous menstruation had been so pain-free.

If spasmodic dysmenorrhoea is bad enough to need regular medication to ease the pain, and especially if it causes the girl to take time off work or stay in bed, then medical help should be sought. It is interesting to listen to mothers explaining why they do not take their daughters to the doctor when they are suffering from spasmodic dysmenorrhoea:

> 'I don't want to be considered fussy or neurotic.'

> 'He will only tell her to get married and have children like I was told!'

> 'I would hate her to have an operation.'

'He might put her on the pill; she's such a nice girl, besides she hasn't any boy-friends yet.'

'Boys would take advantage of her if she were on the pill.'

Such attitudes are a great shame as there is so much that can be done for these girls. If the parents do not want their daughter to have the pill the doctor can always prescribe oestrogen alone, which is not contraceptive but will ease her monthly pains. However, since the introduction of prostaglandin inhibitors, oestrogen and the pill are no longer the only effective treatment.

Even before the onset of the first menstruation cyclical mood swings may occur, and they can continue even at times of missed menstruation (Fig. 6). These mood swings can transform a happy schoolgirl into a lazy, bad-tempered, selfish individual whose academic work and behaviour deteriorate even before menstruation is established. This pattern is very suggestive of the premenstrual syndrome and events should be recorded so that help can be given to the girl before her work falls too far behind her schoolmates'.

During these years one may anticipate marked conflicts between the early maturers and those who mature more slowly. Firm friendships of several years' standing may be broken as one develops and 'fancies herself as a lady' and the other remains a mere schoolgirl. With maturation comes the interest in boys and an appreciation of feminine beauty, so that endless time is spent in caring for her face and body. At this time grease starts developing in the skin and the sweat glands begin to operate, so that skin care and deodorants become necessary.

Many girls do not like the changes in body contour which Nature has decreed: they object to the rounded contours and would prefer the broad shoulders and the gawky limbs of boys. This stimulates the urge to diet, particularly in those who are not even overweight for their height and size. Excessive dieting during these developing years may halt menstruation and ovulation and lead to *anorexia nervosa* which is weight loss accompanied by food phobias and psychological changes. It is not unusual to find girls reducing their weight by strict dieting from nine to five or six stone within a few months, and yet still complaining of their body image and imagining that they are too fat. Unhappily the road to recovery in such cases is slow and halting, and with the development of multicystic ovaries, their future fertility is at stake. Indeed when menstruation does return it is often accompanied by unpleasant premenstrual symptoms.

Unfortunately for most teenagers this sexual development is occurring just at the same time as their mothers are experiencing the difficult years of the menopause and are also subject to mood swings and unpleasant symptoms. Nevertheless it is important to help adolescent girls through this stage, however awkward, impossible and thoughtless they become. They should be given every opportunity to mix freely with both older girls and children, and with boys and men, to help them sort themselves out and appreciate the differences in individual men and women.

At puberty premenstrual depression is usually worse than the tiredness, and is likely to make the girl sullen, secretive, withdrawn and anxious to be alone. Nevertheless, careful observation should be kept of her behaviour as too often the mood swings occur suddenly without warning or provocation and she may make an unexpected suicide gesture.

PHYLLIS, 17 years old, had been captain of her form at 12 years and her work was the envy of others. But she gradually went downhill in work and behaviour. She became slovenly, rude and bored with everything, gave up any attempt at O levels and left school at the first opportunity. She first worked in a hairdresser's shop, but her work was unsatisfactory and her time-keeping poor. Her next job was as a filing clerk, where her work was not appreciated. There would be days when she would come home, slip up to her bedroom and stay there for hours, allowing no one to enter and refusing food. One day her father found her apparently asleep in a corner, but the doctor diagnosed an overdose of hypnotics and arranged for her admission to hospital for a stomach wash-out. This incident so shocked her mother that from then onwards she kept a careful eye on her daughter. Soon the mother noted the correlation of awkwardness and menstruation and asked for medical help. With treatment her daughter brightened up again, restarted her social life which had been absent for five years and later returned to evening classes, obtaining higher qualifications in short-hand and typing.

Girls with premenstrual syndrome deserve treatment in their teens; if progesterone is required it is usually only temporary. Gradually as they mature the need for regular medication passes, although they may need it again at times of stress.

At one British boarding school parents and visitors were invited to inspect the dormitories on the annual Open Day. On the mantelpiece in each of the spotless dormitories was displayed a mark sheet giving the marks each child had received for the tidiness of her bed and locker before going down to breakfast each morning. It was not difficult on inspecting these sheets to determine the menstrual patterns of the girls, for when they were exceptionally sleepy during the premenstruum they were more likely to receive a poor tidiness grade.

At another British boarding school, punishment books were used for recording the names of girls, the date and the reasons for the punishments. These books were made available for analysis together with the books the girls signed when they menstruated and needed sanitary protection. It was found that during menstruation the girls were twice as naughty as would have been expected. Many of the punishments during menstruation were those which could be accounted for by tiredness, and included such offences as forgetfulness and unpunctuality, while others reflected the premenstrual irritability at having to conform to strict school discipline. Indeed, a girl is more likely to be punished for any offence during menstruation as she may be too slow to avoid detection. If several children are all talking when the

teacher enters the classroom, it will be those with a slow
reaction time who will not stop talking quickly enough and
will receive a punishment.

This investigation also showed two types of naughtiness.
When it had been completed the headmistress, an exceptional woman who knew and was concerned with each individual girl, was shown two lists of girls' names and asked to
comment on them. Unknown to her the lists contained the
names of the girls who had received most punishments
during the term. One list contained the names of those whose
punishments had all occurred during the premenstruum.
'Just naughty girls from exuberance or laziness; I'll probably
be choosing a future head girl from that list,' she commented.
But when shown the other list containing the names of girls
whose punishments had occurred evenly throughout the
menstrual cycle she remarked, 'They're the problem girls
requiring careful handling and understanding,' and she went
on to describe how they had to cope with such difficulties
as broken homes, foreign parents, or minor deformities such
as a hare lip.

In this study it was also noted that prefects, girls of 16–18
years, who were permitted to punish girls for misbehaviour,
gave significantly more punishments during their own menstruations, and then their standard gradually fell throughout
the cycle. This naturally raises the problem of teachers, and
indeed of any woman in charge, such as magistrates and
forewomen: do they give more punishments during their
own menstruation? Are they more strict then? Or, once they
appreciate the effect of menstrual hormones on their
behaviour, do they lean over backwards to try to avoid pun-
ishing too severely when they themselves are menstruating?

In this survey it was also possible to analyse how many
days passed before a girl who had been punished once was
punished a second time, a statistical method known as 'critical-event analysis'. The results showed that more second
punishments occurred within four days of the first offence,
then fewer within five to eight days of the first offence, and
so there was a gradual decrease in further punishments until

25–28 days after the first offence when there was an unexpected rise not only in those girls who were already menstruating, but also in girls who had not yet started. This suggests that already these premenarcheal girls were experiencing mood swings, a fact that many observant mothers have already noticed in their daughters. Incidentally it was possible to do a similar analysis in respect of boys at the nearby boarding school, but they did not show evidence of cyclical mood swings.

On one occasion my adolescent daughter burst into the house from school asking for a menstrual chart. When asked why, she replied that her form teacher had lost her temper and thrown a piece of chalk at a girl, and the same thing had occurred on the Thursday before half-term, which was exactly four weeks earlier!

When my daughter left the sixth form she passed on to the next head girl of the school a list, compiled by the girls, of the probable dates of the teachers' menstruation so that the girls would know when to hand in their essays to get good marks.

When, in later years, schoolgirls meet and swop memories it is the unfair incidents and unjustified punishments which are uppermost in their minds. One now wonders how often the blame could have been placed on it being the wrong day of the month for the teachers.

Schoolmistresses have a dual responsibility, not only to cope with their own premenstrual mood swings, but also to recognize the existence of them in the girls for whose education they are responsible. They should be ready to step in with a kind word to girls who appear to have episodes of irritability or become depressed or disheartened, giving encouragement, particularly in preventing a girl from giving up a worthwhile career just because of some minor pinpricks or temporary difficulties of study.

Schoolgirls' work deteriorates during the premenstruum (Fig. 9). A similar survey of girls in the Armed Forces confirmed lower intelligence scores in tests performed by the girls during their paramenstruum.

A study in 1968 into the effect of menstruation on the results of GCE examinations showed that those girls taking examinations during their paramenstruum had fewer passes, fewer distinction marks and a lower average mark. The girls whose results were most affected during the paramenstruum were those with cycles exceeding 31 days and those whose menstruation lasted seven days or longer. In the examinations, some subjects were completed in one day, some had papers four days apart, and other subjects had examination papers at any interval of more than eight days. Consideration of the results in relation to the time intervals between papers on the same subject showed that girls were under greater handicap in those subjects where all papers were completed in one day (when she could be in her paramenstruum) in comparison with subjects where papers were spaced more than eight days apart, in which case the girl could not have been entirely in her paramenstruum during both papers. It should not be difficult for examination boards and universities so to arrange examination timetables that when two papers are necessary for a subject they are eight or more days apart. The GCSE, with its continuous assessment, is aimed at reducing the handicap of menstruation for girls.

It might be mentioned that at public examinations provision is usually made for invigilators to make a note at the top of the examination paper of candidates who are handicapped by the paramenstruum at the time of writing the paper. But it is not known how much notice is taken of this fact by the examiners.

Another hazard is the increased sex desire which may occur premenstrually. This often takes over young adolescents, who are quite unprepared for this new sex urge and unable to control their emotions. This nymphomaniac urge may be responsible for young girls running away from home or custody, only to be found wandering in the park or following the boys. These girls can be helped and their delinquent behaviour abruptly ended with progesterone therapy.

10

Family Life

The word 'marriage' is used within this chapter in its broadest sense 'the union of man and woman as husband and wife' regardless of whether the union was solemnized in a religious ceremony, legalized in a Registry Office, or merely a common decision to live together. This chapter is not concerned with social conventions, but with the impact of premenstrual syndrome on the lives of men, women and children living together as families.

One wonders whether the cynic who wrote 'Marriages are made in heaven, but they end in hell!' was married to a woman who was a severe case of the premenstrual syndrome, or he was just a keen observer of other people's marriages. Of course, not all relationships end up in hell, but when a woman suffers from premenstrual syndrome, or later develops it, the stakes run pretty high. Most men enter relationships sublimely ignorant of the problems women face each month. If their mother or their sister were sufferers they might have learned how to cope with it, but the odds are that they are inclined to think that they are unique in their troubles and really know little about the cause.

Before marriage, and whilst they were going out together, it was easy enough for the woman to conceal those difficult days and all too often it is not until a couple are living together that the awful truth begins to dawn. If she is a sufferer from spasmodic dysmenorrhoea he will be the first to see that she gets good and complete relief of her pains, for pain is something a man can understand. However, sudden mood changes, irrational behaviour, and bursting into tears for no apparent reason are bewildering, while sudden aggression and violence which come with little warning and no justification are deeply disturbing.

Fortunately, not all women suffer from the premenstrual syndrome, nor do all premenstrual syndrome sufferers become hellcats. Even so the male partner should be made aware of the problems that can arise, how to recognize them when they first show themselves, and what treatment is available to provide complete relief. An article in *Bride and Home* described what may lie ahead once the honeymoon is over:

> *'Then quite suddenly you feel as if you can't cope any more – everything seems too much trouble, the endless household chores, the everlasting planning of meals. For no apparent reason you rebel: "Why should I do everything?" you ask yourself defiantly. "I didn't have to do this before I was married. Why should I do it now?" Everything starts going wrong and it gets worse instead of better. As on other mornings you get up and cook breakfast while your husband is in the bathroom. You climb wearily out of bed and trudge down the stairs, a vague feeling of resentment growing within you. The sound of cheerful whistling from upstairs only makes you feel a little more cross. Without any warning the toast starts to scorch and the sausages instead of happily sizzling in the pan start spitting and spluttering furiously. Aghast you rescue the toast which by this time is beyond resurrection and fit only for the bin. The sausages are charred relics of their former selves and you throw those out too. Your unsuspecting husband opens the kitchen door expecting to find his breakfast ready and waiting, only to see a smoky atmosphere and a thoroughly overwrought wife. You are so dismayed at him finding you in such chaos that you just burst helplessly into tears.'*

What is the young husband going to make of that situation? Much depends upon his family background. If he has met similar situations in his home before marriage he will undoubtedly react as he did then, so that if he used to make himself scarce and get out of the house, he'll probably grab his bag and dash for the office leaving his wife to sort out her troubles. If he was in the habit of helping to sort out the chaos, he'll probably sympathize with her, give her a kiss, and make her a cup of coffee and breakfast and insist on her going back to bed for the day. This latter is the wisest course of action.

But what if the young husband has never met this sort of thing. How will he cope? Will he shrug it off hoping that it is only a temporary lapse until, once a month, month after month, it recurs? Or will he rage about breakfast being ruined and storm out of the house to arrive at work hungry and unable to do his work properly, eventually returning home in a tired and frustrated state to an equally distraught wife? Not a happy augury for the future.

So far, in this chapter, we've been considering the state of a young couple affected by premenstrual syndrome. There are those who don't start their symptoms until after a pregnancy. Just think of the situation. For a year or more they've been enjoying an idyllic life together until the baby comes along and now once a month there are frustrations, mood swings, irritability, and apparent laziness in addition to coping with the baby. The man may find that now he can do nothing right on those terrible days. If he has been sensible and kept a diary of her menstrual dates he will soon recognize the time relationship and, realizing the importance of frequent starchy snacks for those with premenstrual syndrome, will keep a careful eye on her eating habits.

On the other hand if he hasn't been sensible, if neither he nor she have any clear idea of her menstrual dates, they'll probably go on month after month until he can stand it no longer.

But all this suffering is quite unnecessary and a tragic destruction of family life. The answer to it lies in the ability of a husband and wife to share equally in every aspect of their lives. If they both keep a menstrual chart of her menstruation and any symptoms that she may have, they will soon realize when things are going wrong and then is the time to seek medical advice and obtain treatment for it. If, together, they keep the chart it will help them to understand each other better and the man will have a much greater understanding of what menstruation means to a woman. He will also find that he is the first to notice the warning signs of premenstrual syndrome. The slight irrationality of her conversation, or lack of conversation, the minor disagreements in which there is a certain rigidity in her views. More important still is the darkening of the skin around her eyes, one of the surest signs that she is about to enter her premenstruum. In some women the skin goes so dark as to appear almost black.

If there are children he should remember that they are more likely to get out of hand with Mother no longer able to care for and play with them. He must try to be a substitute mother as well as a father and exercise his control over them. He should remember that there is housework to be done and it is no use telling her to rest, he has to be practical. If the work has to be done and there is no one else to do it, she will not rest. A neighbour or a relative could be asked to help; it will probably only be for four or five days, unless it is very severe. Once menstruation has started, and while events are still fresh in their minds, he should impress upon her the need for medical help and assure her that he will go with her. More husbands accompany their wives to the doctor or hospital when seeking help for premenstrual syndrome than for any other gynaecological condition, and this includes infertile couples seeking help.

The following quotes from recent mail reveal how often the husband is implicated in the premenstrual syndrome:

> *'I am fortunate in having an extremely long-suffering husband who puts up with my tirades as best he knows how, but he says he doesn't know how to cope with me.'*

*'My husband first noticed the connection with my men-
strual cycle without mentioning it to me eighteen months
ago, and backs me up completely in writing to you.'*

*'The misery has gone on for years, misery and misery.
Seventeen jobs in ten years. Now I clean offices, and for
two weeks out of the month my husband gets up at 4.00
a.m. and does them for me.'*

Not uncommonly the husbands have devised their own
means of confirming beforehand; thus the computer pro-
grammer came complete with a computer printout to prove
it, while a draughtsman turned up with a beautifully drawn
blueprint; others merely bring along the office diary or
kitchen calendar.

But there are still too many husbands who have not made
the diagnosis or, more rarely, do not realize that help is
available. They may know when they wake up that it's one
of those days and no matter what they do, they will not be
able to satisfy her. If he returns home with some red roses
she'll ask, 'Why didn't you bring me my favourite chocolates?' but when he brings the correct brand of chocolates
it'll be, 'You know I'm dieting, how very cruel of you.' He
just can't win.

The monthly problems may interfere with his social life
and his earning capacity. Some years ago a door-to-door
salesman was sent by his employer for medical help. He
worked on a commission basis, and whilst his average commission was £80 per week, in one week in four the sum fell
to something nearer £20. Not only did he find it difficult
to plan to make ends meet financially, but his chances of
promotion were affected. The salesman explained that he
became more depressed and seemed to start work later
during the weeks his earnings were low. When asked about
his wife's menstruation the significance dawned on him. A
few days later he brought along his wife's menstrual record
which confirmed the diagnosis. Her irritability and tiredness
were hindering her husband. She was delighted to be offered

progesterone treatment and responded well. Her husband
was also delighted when he got promotion.

Marital disharmony is a recurring theme among those seeking medical help:

> 'My marriage broke up seven years ago and I feel this
> trouble was a big cause of the break-up. I have since turned
> down a chance to remarry as I cannot face burdening some-
> one with my continual monthly ailments.'

> 'This premenstrual misery is a very real threat to the sur-
> vival of our marriage.'

> 'We have been married for eight years during which time
> my premenstrual tension has been a constant problem.
> During the past three years this has become more acute
> and increasingly more severe with traumatic effect on our
> relationship and that of our two boys of five and three
> years.'

> 'My husband has urged me to write; our marriage is break-
> ing up, my children are suffering and after five years of
> my trouble my poor husband can take no more.'

> 'My husband has already left me and I have two children
> whom I try hard not to lose my temper with at this time,
> but I feel sorry for them, it is really awful.'

> 'I have come to dread my periods and even my husband
> rushes to the calendar at an unexpected outburst on my
> part. I get violent with my husband.'

Sometimes the disharmony shows as just silence. On other
occasions there are vicious verbal battles, and at the extreme
limit there are the fights and batterings. How many wives
batter their husbands during their paramenstruum is
unknown, or how often the husband is provoked beyond
endurance and batters her.

One mother wrote about her daughter who was receiving treatment for premenstrual irritability and food cravings:

'Some cakes and biscuits disappeared on Sunday. It was all too much for me and I burst into tears. This in turn upset my husband, who went and found Mary in her bedroom and gave her a good thrashing. At midnight we discovered she was missing. She had spent the night with friends. Both Mary and I started menstruating that day.'

Here is a case of menstrual synchrony, with mother's and daughter's menstruation occurring at the same time and where the mother's tears caused the fraught husband to beat his daughter.

Two researchers from Washington, Roger Langley and Richard Levy, have estimated that there are 12 million battered husbands in the United States. They reckon it is the 'most unreported crime', affecting 20% of husbands. Again one is just left wondering on the effect of the paramenstruum, how often were the battering wives victims of their own hormonal imbalance?

A couple of quotes to suggest that the premenstruum may frequently by the cause:

'I attacked him with a carving knife on one occasion, and whilst building a stone wall I lifted huge stones and hurled them at him.'

'I have tried to knife my husband too many times to count . . . but for one fantastic week I feel on top of the world.'

Most marriage-guidance counsellors are well versed in the traumas which can be caused to the marital relationship by the premenstrual syndrome and try to draw the partner's attention to this. The wise counsellors, when telephoned urgently for help because of a massive quarrel, will arrange a meeting seven days later when the woman is more likely to be in her rational postmenstrual phase, having more insight and being more amenable to reason.

While a wife may be content for most of the month coping with the cooking, cleaning, shopping, mending, ironing, and perhaps even the gardening, there may come one of those days when it all gets on top of her, when she's too apathetic to cope with everyday chores, when she burns the cooking, and leaves the house untidy and in a slovenly condition. Alternatively she may have a spurt of restless energy, obsessionally polishing all and sundry until she wears herself out and then blames her premenstrual symptoms on the fact that she 'overdid it'. The busier she is the quicker time passes and the longer the intervals between food. One difficulty facing the housewife at home all day is the temptation to miss meals, waiting to enjoy an evening meal with her husband at night. During the paramenstruum she will be facing the problems of low blood sugar levels.

The working wife faces different problems. In her effort to control herself in front of her workmates, and possibly also the public, she stores up her problems until she reaches home and then lets rip at her nearest and dearest. Again she may well have missed her lunch and gone a long interval without food, not appreciating the problems this causes.

A most important problem the couple must face will be that of sexual harmony. Dr Ruth D'arcy Hart found that among married women 60% found their sex urge was greatest before menstruation, but unfortunately for those with the premenstrual syndrome this is also the time at which many of them are most horrible to their partners, and when to spite him she refuses his sexual overtures. It is the time when it is so easy for her to claim she's too tired. Incidentally, one of the side effects of the pill is its ability to decrease the natural sex urge. Satisfactory sex between partners is the best cement for any relationship. There is so much that can be done these days, if difficulties develop on this side of a relationship, that it is worthwhile seeking help. One cause of the decrease in sexual satisfaction, which has only recently been recognized but is more responsive to treatment, is a loss of sex urge occurring after a pregnancy complicated by postnatal depression. A blood test may show the wife to have a raised prolactin level in which case treatment with bromocriptine can be effective.

Men do not have cycles akin to women. On page 90 a 'critical-event analysis' is described which detected cycles of naughtiness in premenarcheal girls. A similar one has also been done in various surveys of behaviour in relation to men and prisoners, schoolboys and symptoms of glaucoma. The results were similar: there appeared to be a return of the critical event after an interval of 25–28 days in women but not in men.

Margaret Henderson of Australia claims that men have a similar ovulation temperature chart which is synchronous with the wife's chart. When she has her mid-cycle temperature drop, followed by a rise after ovulation lasting for 12 to 14 days until she menstruates, the husband also has a temperature drop and rise, but the temperature rise is only maintained for 2–5 days. When the wife has an anovular cycle, or goes on the pill, the husband may also stop cycling, or more commonly, he may cycle alone with a much shorter cycle length. If his wife is pregnant and stops ovulating, Henderson suggests that the man may harmonize in the same way, for babies have been born at the end of a father's cycle. However, the number of men studied was small and there is very little supporting evidence available.

As mentioned earlier a good proportion of partners will attend at the surgery with the woman if she is suffering from the premenstrual syndrome and the remainder will usually agree to come together at the next interview. This is a most valuable opportunity to learn more of the full extent of the wife's problems. At the same time there is much useful information which can be given to the husband to help him cope better with the situation. First he must understand what premenstrual syndrome is, why it occurs, and the importance of the dietary regime. He should appreciate which of his wife's many symptoms can be helped and which are not premenstrual, but occurring throughout the month, and therefore not likely to benefit from progesterone treatment. He should be taught how to chart the symptoms, and may like to keep his own chart of events. Often the husband is the first to appreciate that his wife could benefit by some extra progesterone, and if she is receiving it by suppositories it is usually possible to give him full permission to raise the dose when he feels the need is there. The husband should also appreciate the problems of low blood sugar levels, and that his wife will be worse if deprived of sleep. He should also appreciate that during the premenstruum her desire for alcohol will increase but she will also become intoxicated more easily, possibly on half her usual amount.

If the husband fully understands the situation he will be able to make the necessary adjustments to their life. Thus one husband, realizing his wife's irritability in the premenstruum, asked the bank manager to send their joint balance sheets on specified days so that they could discuss their financial arrangements calmly in her postmenstruum. During the premenstruum when the wife has little insight, many decisions like moving, holidays and schools must either be taken by the husband or postponed for a week or so until rational discussions are a possibility. If help in the home is needed it may be better to arrange this for the one vital week of the month rather than merely one day per week.

How much responsibility should a husband have for his wife's premenstrual violence? In addition to ensuring that she receives treatment from her doctor, and making provision for the care of the children and the home when she is at her most vulnerable, does he have a responsibility for the protection of the public? Should he report her violence to some appropriate authority? and indeed, which is the appropriate authority? What are his responsibilities if her violence brings her to court in conflict with criminal law? Too often such cases are reported too late, when the woman is already in the dock having pleaded guilty to a charge of assault, infanticide, or murder, and the husband in her defence will produce disturbing stories of her cyclical problems. All these questions need serious consideration, for at the present time there is no clear guidance available to help the unfortunate husband in such desperate circumstances.

11

Menfolk

Premenstrual syndrome is a man's problem too. With some 40% of women suffering from premenstrual syndrome, the law of averages means that sooner or later the man will find himself on the receiving end. It could be his mother, sister, partner, girl-friend, a woman in his workplace or anywhere else. If he has not learned to handle the situation and does not know where to get help, it can be very traumatic indeed.

It has often been said that if men suffered from premenstrual syndrome they would soon have found a cure. Well, men do suffer from the effects of premenstrual syndrome among the women with whom they come into contact either at work or play. This has been the case for thousands of years, yet men are mighty slow at recognizing it, diagnosing it and understanding the treatment required. Those men who do suffer rarely talk about it to other men and therefore feel they are dealing with an exceptional, unpredictable or difficult woman. When they do talk to other men they are surprised to find that many have similar problems, and that some men are even worse off.

Male Reaction
Only those who have encountered the sudden personality change of a woman severely affected by premenstrual syndrome, and have come face to face with an unreasonable and

angry virago of a woman, will have any idea of the trauma and sense of unreality experienced by the man. As the emotion of this irrational situation sweeps away common sense and reason, a feeling of numbness takes over and his thinking becomes disjointed and incoherent; he feels powerless and immobilized by the torrent of vituperation that submerges his own personality, until he flees in confusion and desperation.

This situation is graphically presented in the introduction to David Duff's book *Albert and Victoria*, which portrays the reaction of Prince Albert, Lord Melbourne and the cabinet minister. He vividly describes their confusion and inability to cope when faced with an irrational outburst of premenstrual syndrome from the Queen, whose tension, irritability, changing moods, violence and periods of negative attitudes were quite incomprehensible. All three were left baffled, unsure of what they should do and quite unable to deal effectively with the situation.

Albert, the Prince Consort, was perplexed. His reaction was to try logical arguments. Like many other men, he did not appreciate or understand the unreasoned emotion in Queen Victoria's brain. He didn't realize that you can't talk logic to the illogical mind of a premenstrual syndrome sufferer.

Even Lord Melbourne, 'a past master at dealing with women', was quite unable to deal with this situation. The poor cabinet minister fled in disarray, too frightened even to observe the protocol of retirement from the royal presence. Here were three men, presumably of the highest intelligence, so severely affected by premenstrual syndrome that they were unable to take any positive action or do anything to prevent a recurrence.

Ten years earlier, Charles Lamb, the English essayist, had died. For some twenty-five years he was at the receiving end of recurrent attacks of premenstrual violence from his sister, Mary Lamb, during one of which she killed her mother. Each month at the time of her premenstrual violence, with her consent, he locked her up in a special closet. With great

loyalty and courage Charles took upon himself the burden
of responsibility for her care. He was rewarded with her
lifelong and affectionate devotion, keeping house for him
and helping with his writings, which demonstrates her postmenstrual normality.

Similar events are occurring daily yet most turn a blind
eye to them. Is it not time that menfolk decided to learn
more about this disease and the way to handle it? It has been
suggested that it is a disease of twentieth-century civilization,
but this is only true to the extent that the media today exploits
it and it offers fair pickings for quacks and entrepreneurs.

Premenstrual syndrome has been around for thousands of
years. Hippocrates, in 400BC, reacted with a logical explanation. He suggested that it was due to the 'agitated blood
trying to find a way out of the body'. A century earlier
Simonides of Ceos, the Greek poet, wrote a classic poem
about the changing moods of women, which he likened to
the changing moods of the sea. This provides an unmistak-
able representation of the sudden personality changes of the
premenstrual woman.

Men are Different

'Why can't a woman behave like a man?' explodes Professor
Higgins in Bernard Shaw's *Pygmalion* and Lowe's *My Fair
Lady*. Thousands of men must have felt like this when faced
with the effects of their fair lady's premenstrual syndrome.
Professor Higgins's outburst can be taken in two ways – as
frustrated protest or as a serious question. Nature having
planned males and females for different functions in reproduction has also ensured that a woman cannot behave like
a man, nor a man behave like a woman. Men and women
are different but equal. What is more, it is impossible for a
man to go through what a woman has to go through as a
consequence of her role in Nature's plan. A healthy man has
no idea of how it feels for those few women with serious
premenstrual syndrome who are unable to control their
actions or behaviour at certain times of the month. Men need

to be aware of these women's problems, and be sympathetic and supportive during these premenstrual days. They should realize and reassure her that help is available and that there is no reason for a woman to suffer unnecessarily. Now the hormonal background of premenstrual syndrome is becoming increasingly understood, there is so much more that can be done to control and eliminate this suffering.

Recognize the Early Signs

Some men are unaware of the problem until they awake one morning to find that their partner has become a hysterical and completely irrational woman with whom it is impossible to reason and who may become violent. This is recognizing premenstrual syndrome the hard way. Others, who are more observant, may gradually become aware of their partner's changing moods. She may become pessimistic, negative, withdrawn and difficult to please. She may be snappy, argumentative, impatient, illogical and irrational. She may shout, shriek, yell, swear or become completely hysterical. She may even be violent, ready to bang the table, slam doors, throw plates, vases, books, kick the dog or cat or hit her nearest and dearest, which means her partner and her children.

Not every sufferer of premenstrual syndrome knows she has got the disease. She may have accepted her failings as part of her explosive personality, and something that cannot be changed.

During her premenstruum she may change her likes and dislikes of food, clothes or furnishings. She may have food binges, alcoholic urges or spending sprees, buying things she does not need, clothes that do not fit and food she never eats.

Some women have 'lazy' days when they'd rather not exert themselves. Others have 'energetic' days, when they won't sit down and are for ever tidying up and finding more jobs to do. Yet others have 'urgent' days when everything must be done today immediately, not tomorrow or next week. No two women are alike.

A few women become paranoid during the premenstruum, and will accuse their partner of all sorts of outrageous behaviour, often suspecting an affair. These are the 'unforgetting' and 'unforgiving' days, which will pass. Some women have 'jealousy' days, which recur monotonously each cycle. Until the woman is treated, these days have to be accepted. Her partner can help by trying not to show any interest in other women.

How to Cope

The most important piece of advice during the woman's difficult time is don't reason, discuss or argue with her. Above all keep control of yourself, and try hard not to be argumentative or angry. Try not to say 'Of course! it's the wrong time of the month'; or to show her the menstrual chart which will prove you are right. Do keep assuring her of your concern, support and love. She needs this, even though she may reject it. Especially try to help her to eat little and often. Find her favourite snacks and make sure there are plenty around for her to pick up and nibble. Don't worry if she has an eating binge. It is a sign that the sugar stores in her body are seriously depleted and she needs to replenish them. Instead make sure she can eat some starchy food every three hours. There's more about that in Chapter 20 (pages 196–8). Discourage her from starting a weight loss diet until her premenstrual syndrome has been properly treated. Admire her good qualities, but don't mention her weight, or tease her about her figure. If necessary phone her to ensure she is eating regularly, or ask a neighbour to pop in. If she has a taste for alcohol, she may well have uncontrollable alcohol urges during this time, so keep an eye on the home supplies and if they are going down too rapidly remove all alcohol from the house.

Explain to the children that Mother is not well today. If possible arrange for a neighbour, friend, or member of the family to care for them for a day or even a few hours. Opportunities will always occur to repay the kindness at another time. Children can also be very helpful in ensuring that Mother eats regularly if given the necessary instructions, but leave the food in a convenient place.

Use these difficult days to learn the true facts about premenstrual syndrome. Make an appointment to see her doctor in the postmenstruum. Doctors are often more sympathetic to premenstrual syndrome when the partner accompanies the patient. Remember to take the menstrual chart with you: it is the only thing the doctor needs to make a firm diagnosis. Tell the doctor how it is affecting your life as well as hers. Find out about local support and self-help groups. Many support groups encourage partners, and if your group does, take advantage of it. Many men are surprised at the severe suffering others have to endure.

When peace and tranquillity returns in the postmenstruum show her the menstrual chart you have been keeping, and discuss the implications. Have a heart to heart discussion, and emphasize that you now understand why it has all happened. Encourage her to see her doctor, and, most importantly, remind her that there is satisfactory treatment available. If possible, discuss the importance of the three-hourly starchy diet and start with it straightaway, remembering that it must be rigidly adhered to every day of the month.

If it is necessary to give her progesterone treatment, learn all about it, and see that she takes it as instructed. If the woman is allowed to increase the dose when needed, the man is usually the first to realize when it is best for her to do so. If she is a candidate for progesterone injections, he should consider whether he can give them. It is not a difficult task.

When men have learned to recognize premenstrual syndrome and how to help sufferers there will be no need for them to be on the receiving end. Harmony will be returned to the household, and women will be happier and more able to cope with their lives.

12

Mother

The mother is the lynchpin of the family. When her life becomes a misery each month, because of the disturbances of the premenstrual syndrome, the consequences affect the whole family: husband, infants, schoolchildren and teenagers. Children, even infants of only a few months, are sensitive to changes in the mother's temperament, and because they cannot understand the reason, they react to it in their own peculiar way.

When you ask adult sufferers of the premenstrual syndrome if their mother also suffered in the same way, you are likely to get many positive, and some interesting, replies, such as:

> *'We used to say "The dragon's on the warpath" and we all knew what it meant. But it only lasted a day or two.'*

> *'I remember my brother putting up a red flag outside the front door to warn us to be careful in our approach to Mother.'*

Health visitors and social workers soon recognize when one of the mothers in their care is in her premenstruum. The usually tidy house is slovenly and disorganized, the carpets littered with old clothes, dirty dishes still on the kitchen table and probably a burnt cake by the sink. Maybe the children went off to school late, and in yesterday's togs, and the chances are that the meals will not be ready in time.

Although premenstrual syndrome may start at puberty it usually gets worse, or it can begin, after the children are born, especially if there has been any depression after childbirth; this was a recurring theme in many letters:

'Since the birth of my last child two years ago (I have five children) I have changed from being a perfectly normal housewife and mother to an unpredictable bad-tempered person. During my period my moods make me feel positively ill, especially my head. If only I could grow a new one I say to my husband.'

'I have had intervals of depression since the birth of my first child so that I have never regained confidence in myself since then.'

'After the baby's birth I changed and now I get an incredible amount of head pressure for a few days prior to the bleeding. It was as though the top of my head was about to blow off with pressure. I spoke to my doctor about the possibility of my starting an early menopause but he only smiled, and said it was more likely premenstrual tension.'

'I have a twenty-two-month-old son and I cannot remember feeling like this before he was born. I do love him very much but the poor little soul does have a terrible time when I shout at him and make him sob his heart out and I seem unable to stop although I feel terrible about what I'm doing. It is almost as though I must be getting some sort of pleasure from it, and I feel very, very upset and guilty afterwards.'

Dr Christine Cooper, a paediatrician, has stated that children can also be psychologically damaged for life by verbal violence.

The sudden onset of irritability after the birth of a child is a cause of surprise to many mothers, who did not experience it before. They suddenly find themselves becoming quick-tempered, and making totally irrational decisions. They become impatient with the children, not waiting for them to learn to dress or eat for themselves. They won't accept that 'kids will be kids' and shout at them when they are romping about harmlessly and then complain that the children won't behave. They are like the school prefects who expect a higher standard of discipline when they themselves are menstruating.

When Mother's got so much to do it's easy enough to miss out meals, which always has the additional benefit of slimming her too. Unfortunately her irritable and aggressive outbursts are likely to occur when her blood sugar level is at its lowest, which makes matters even worse.

> ROSE, an intelligent unmarried mother of 24 years, had contacted the NSPCC herself as she feared she might harm her six-year-old son during her premenstruum. It was obvious from her story that she had been very near to damaging him. She then described the usual timetable for the day, 'getting up at 8.00 a.m. and having a meal of toast and coffee together and then walking half a mile to his school, doing the shopping on the way home, housework until it was time to fetch him from the school at 3.30 p.m.' This was the worst time of the day and just before her periods she would feel aggressive as she met him; suddenly a surge of hatred would well up and if he didn't behave, this was the time he would be smacked.

In fact, Rose was describing how she became irritable with her son 7½ hours after her last meal, having been energetic during the interval. Her menstrual chart confirmed that she only lost her temper during the premenstruum, and since having treatment with progesterone and eating a midday meal she has been happier and trouble free. Incidentally, Rose would mark in advance on her menstrual chart the days on which she had to exert extra self-control as she was so anxious to do all that was best for her son.

Two remarks often heard after successful treatment of these parents is 'Even my children behave better' and 'They don't shout so much nowadays'. Some doctors even write in their files 'CBB' meaning 'children behaving better'. In fact, the children respond quicker to their mother's improved temper than do the family pets, which have been kicked. Animals take a long time to forget.

Contraception often proves a problem for these mothers. Those with the premenstrual syndrome are liable to have side effects on the pill. Intra-uterine devices can cause increased oestrogen production, resulting in heavy menstruation becoming even heavier. Unfortunately tubal ligation, previously thought to be a convenient and permanent solution, has been shown to reduce the progesterone blood level. If they are receiving progesterone this can be used contraceptively, as discussed on pages 217–18.

Children Cannot Understand

Children, who cannot understand the mood swings in their mothers, may react with the development of psychosomatic or bodily symptoms, such as a cough, runny nose, endless crying, temper tantrums or vomiting. In my general practice, when children attended with such complaints the mother would be given a chart on which to record the dates of the child's symptoms and another one for the mother to record the dates of her own menstruation. When the mother returned with the charts after an interval of two or three months it is surprising how often it was clearly shown that the child was reacting, with various ailments, to the mother's mood swings. A survey of 100 mothers attending surgery because their child had a cough or cold showed that 54% of the mothers were in their paramenstruum. Those children who were brought in during the mother's paramenstruum had a tendency to be under two years; only children; those with symptoms of less than 24-hour duration; and those whose mothers were under 30 years of age. One girl was only nine months, yet her mother brought a chart showing that each time she had menstruated in the previous three months the child had developed a cough and runny nose.

A six-month-old girl was brought to the survey with herpes (or shingles) on her knee, by her mother who had recurrent premenstrual herpes on her upper lip of several years' duration.

A further survey was carried out among children who were admitted as emergencies to the North Middlesex Hospital. The mothers of 100 children were interviewed, and the result was very similar; in fact 49% of the mothers were in their paramenstruum on the day the child was admitted. Some were admitted because of an illness such as asthma, abdominal pain, or a temperature of unknown cause, while others had been injured in an accident. If the mother is accident prone during her paramenstruum, the child she is looking after is also accident prone. If the mother is tired during the paramenstruum she will not notice little Johnny running into an oncoming car or climbing a dangerous tree, and so even he will be in greater danger then.

One day a telephone call informed me that an 18-month-old boy had had a high temperature and a convulsion. This was the third convulsion at intervals of three to four weeks. Enquiry revealed that it was not related to the mother's menstrual cycle, but to the Nanny, who had total care of the boy while the mother worked full-time. There had been some trouble with Nanny the day before and she had been given notice. The two previous convulsions had occurred at the time of Nanny's paramenstruum.

Sibling Jealousy

Sometimes jealousy of a brother or sister is incorrectly diagnosed, when the real diagnosis is premenstrual syndrome in the mother.

SUSAN, aged 30 years, had been very well during her second pregnancy, with plenty of energy so that she would take three-year-old David out each afternoon to play on the swings or kick a football in the nearby recreation park. She had an easy delivery of a much wanted daughter, but afterwards became so depressed that she needed psychiatric treatment. David had been dry since the age of sixteen months, but after his sister's birth he gradually started to wet the bed again, not every night, but in batches every few weeks. It seemed all too easy to blame it on to jealousy of the new baby, but when the mother kept a careful record it showed that David's bedwetting was occurring during the mother's premenstruum. Mother then agreed she 'hadn't been the same' since the baby's birth, and had been too tired and busy to take David out for his usual playtime in the park.

Battered Children

The most tragic presentation of premenstrual syndrome is when it reaches such severity that the mother, in a state of confusion and rage, batters her much loved child. These mothers, contrary to popular belief, are women who really love their child; they have strong maternal feelings, but in a sudden moment of premenstrual irritability their control is lost and they injure their darling child.

A social worker's report on a 35-year-old mother of two children reads:

'During the last premenstruum her youngest daughter, aged 18 months, was screaming and would not stop. Patient was very irritated by this and picked her up and squeezed her – this started a circle of louder screaming and harder squeezing until the patient "heard something crack". She was immediately frightened and threw the child on the floor and sat crying on the chair. When more composed she examined Joan and took her to the doctor.'

This type of injury to a child is not uncommon, judging by the letters and confidences of patients; it suggests that the cases of baby-battering that are coming to light are only the tip of an iceberg.

> 'Because I lost my temper and hit my eldest child when he was four, just before a period, I nearly had a complete nervous breakdown. Even though I feel much better now my premenstrual tension remains and from day 18 of the cycle until day 4 of my period I suffer from depression, temper, forgetfulness and dizziness. It has got to a stage now that every month something the children do triggers me off. It is as though there is somebody inside saying terrible things. I blame my son and tell him I hate him and hit him. Sometimes he gets out of my way quickly.'

If the situation deteriorates the children may be taken into care, but this is a drastic step. One is left wondering about the after-effects of the many slightly battered children, those who are not spotted by the social services and are not helped. Does the unsettled temperamental background of childhood leave any marks such as shyness or lack of confidence?

A woman, who had been treated with progesterone for seventeen years, was asked if she would like to take part in a television commentary dealing with premenstrual syndrome. She went home and explained to her family that she couldn't recall those far-off days. 'By Jove – Dad and I will never be able to forget your vicious temper,' was the comment by the daughter, now in her twenties.

A 35-year-old teacher, married to a headmaster, stated:

> 'For seven days during the premenstruum I became tense, irritable, shouting, weepy and tired, bloated with swelling of my legs and ankles and with headaches over my eyes. I have two children and at those times when I am in an uncontrollable temper I have hit them really hard.'

She was successfully treated with progesterone for twelve

months and has been free from symptoms since. She later wrote:

> 'It has been a valuable experience – I would never have believed that an intelligent woman like me, with high morals and good education, could ever lose control of herself to such an extent that she would batter her children, for I love my children dearly. How utterly illogical it is that I personally should cause them permanent harm.'

When the child reaches school the teacher may notice that absences seem to be occurring at regular intervals. One ten-year-old girl was referred for treatment by her teacher who noticed absences for a few days at the beginning of each month. The teacher, in fact, wondered if it was because of the girl's menstruation, but it transpired that Mother had recurrent premenstrual asthma requiring rest in bed and the daughter was kept at home to answer the door.

Teenagers' Reactions

Playing truant from school may also occur, as in the case of one mother who wrote:

> 'For days before a period starts I hate everyone and make the family's life a misery. My thirteen-year-old daughter will not go to school when I'm like this. She is frightened of what I will do and cries when I start drinking.

Teenagers, both boys and girls, are quick enough to spot the changes in their mother and notice when she's 'in one of those moods' or as one boy said, 'Our whole life revolves around Mom's periods.'

The mother's problem is not helped when the daughter starts to menstruate if they both occur together in synchrony. Many mothers, recognizing the problem in themselves, initially seek help for their daughter's premenstrual syndrome, believing that as they've weathered the storm so far it won't be long before the end. However, they are not prepared to let their daughters suffer as they have done.

Finally, all mothers, and fathers too, have the responsibility of seeing that their children get good sex education, and especially to know about those problems which can come back once a month.

13

The World's Workers

The cost to industry of menstrual problems is high, and it is measured in millions of pounds, lira, kroner, or dollars and not in terms of human misery, unhappiness or pain. It has been estimated to cost British industry 3% of its total wage bill, which may be compared with 3% in Italy, 5% in Sweden and 8% in America. The load is not spread evenly, for the industries which suffer most are those employing large numbers of women, especially the clothing industry, light engineering, transistor and assembly factories and laundries. Texas Instruments, which employs women for the assembly of electrical components, finds that the average worker's normal production rate of 100 components per hour drops during the paramenstruum to 75 per hour.

Research studies have shown that during the paramenstruum there is a deterioration of arm and head steadiness, which is an adverse factor among those whose work demands manual dexterity. One chiropodist complained that during the paramenstruum her hands got stiff and she found skilled movements difficult. 'If ever I do cut a patient you can be sure it will be during those premenstrual days.' One wonders if the same ever applies to surgeons.

Absenteeism, directly from menstrual problems, is generally due to spasmodic dysmenorrhoea, premenstrual migraine and asthma for, as one library assistant remarked, 'You don't stay away from work merely because of your bad temper, instead you soldier on and cause chaos by misfiling, and you get yourself a bad name.' The influence of menstrual illness during working hours was demonstrated in a survey at a light engineering factory in North London employing 3,500 women and also in the branches of a multiple store employing 10,000 women. It showed that 45% of the 269 women reporting sick were in their paramenstruum. In America, Bickers and Woods, as long ago as 1951, noted that 36% of women in their premenstrual week requested sedation during working hours.

Twenty years ago a survey in four London hospitals showed that half of all emergency admissions to hospitals occurred during the premenstruum and these findings have since been confirmed worldwide. This figure was the same for the medical emergencies, like coronaries and strokes, for the surgical admissions like colic and appendicitis, for infectious fevers and for admission to the psychiatric wards. Admissions for depression and attempted suicides have been shown the world over to be the highest during the paramenstruum.

Accidents at work are another problem to industry, both the minor cuts and bruises, which are a waste of working time and are treated at the sick bay, and the serious ones admitted to hospital. Research at the US Center for Safety Education showed that the 48 hours before the onset of menstruation are the most dangerous ones when most accidents at work occur. In Germany it was noted that apprentice tightrope walkers had most accidents in the premenstruum. In restaurants it is recognized that the premenstrual clumsiness of waitresses accounts for an undue number of breakages.

The lowering of mental ability during the paramenstruum accounts for unnecessary typing errors and more than one secretary has been referred for treatment when her boss could no longer put up with those few days in each month when letters had to be returned for retyping. Journalists, artists and authors find this a problem too, lacking inspiration and waiting hopefully for a brainwave, which is more likely to come during the postmenstruum. Errors of billing, accounts, stocktaking and filing take longer to correct than to perform, and again the incidence of mistakes is highest during the paramenstruum. Premenstrual irritability may show itself in bad-tempered service by shopworkers, receptionists and waitresses, who are in the public eye. Lowered judgement during the premenstruum must also be considered by teachers, magistrates and examiners. Hasty and wrong decisions are the problems of the executives. One teacher wrote with honesty, 'Every month there are one or two days when I am simply not worth the salary my employers pay me.'

There are some specialized occupations which would appear to have their own particular hazards on those premenstrual days, such as the hoarseness which affects opera and other professional singers. One musical-comedy star in the 1930s would, with devastating regularity, come into the theatre once a month surrounded by a powerful aroma of garlic which preceded her wherever she went. 'You see,' she would explain, 'it's this sore throat again and garlic is the only thing that saves my voice.' Sure enough four days later she would once again be in magnificent voice, but whether it was the garlic or her postmenstruum that was responsible is a matter for guesswork. For artists in the theatre premenstrual syndrome is a very real problem. One great impresario/producer would always attend rehearsal wearing a top hat and smoking a cigar. On one occasion his leading lady was making heavy weather of it and was obviously in her premenstruum. The great man stood up in the centre of the auditorium, ground his cigar to dust under his feet and hurling his hat on the floor stamped on it crying out, 'Woman! I don't know why I employ you, you drive me to distraction!' There was a pause and in a changed voice he went on, 'But when you are well – you're magnificent!'

One wonders how many of the so-called 'prima donnas' with their reputations for throwing tantrums were really only reacting to their premenstrual syndrome? For the members of the chorus, the showgirls and ballet dancers it is always a question of whether the stage manager has enough experience to realize their problem and help them over those difficult days. Their problems of bloatedness, puffy eyes and skin are also shared by models and film stars who often have a clause in their contracts forbidding filming during the paramenstruum. The lowered sensitivity to taste is a handicap to cooks, who may overflavour the sauces and other foods. Nor must we forget the woman astronaut, Russia's Valentina Tereshkova, who in 1973 had to be brought down after only three days in space when she began to menstruate heavily in the zero gravity.

In Argentina, by constitution, women are allowed to take the necessary days off for their menstrual miseries, and in India wives have long had the privilege of being excused housework as it is known that any food they prepare may be spoilt.

The site of an individual's premenstrual symptoms may be determined by her work. An investigation into the incidence of the premenstrual syndrome was carried out in a light engineering factory. About twenty women were interviewed in batches each day. Some days it was noted that the predominant symptom was premenstrual backache, and on other days headache was the commonest symptom. Later it transpired that all the women in any one batch came from the same department and were doing the same kind of work. Those who spent their working hours stooped over a workbench were more likely to complain of backache, while those employed sitting at a bench assembling minute electrical parts, a task needing considerable mental concentration, were mostly those complaining of premenstrual headaches.

Texas Instruments found that women had less menstrual absenteeism when they worked from 2 p.m. to 10 p.m. compared with the other shifts of 6 a.m. to 2 p.m. and 8.30 a.m. to 5.30 p.m. Maybe this was because the woman who woke up feeling ill had more time to dose herself and recover from her problems. It is certainly a point worth considering by those who are given an option for choosing their own working hours. Sufferers of the premenstrual syndrome usually cope especially badly with night-shift work, which seems to be because the 'Diurnal Clock', which determines the hours of sleep and wakefulness, is situated in the hypothalamus and it easily disturbs the menstrual clock. This has been found to be a problem with nurses, especially those in training whose regulations demand a specified period of night work. Night work too often leads to upsets of the menstrual pattern and to depressive illnesses in sufferers of premenstrual syndrome.

Premenstrual syndrome can affect the chances of getting employment, holding the job down, receiving promotion and losing it unnecessarily.

The problems of some sufferers are shown in the following quotations from letters:

> 'I cannot plan to go anywhere during these depressing times and I live in constant fear of losing my job as I have to take time off each month with a real sick headache. My chances of promotion have been ruined because of this.'

> 'I have recently thrown up my job unnecessarily and realized that it is ridiculous to let this condition ruin my whole life. Although I know the cause of my depressive feelings I seem to be unable to think logically and though I know I shall be fine again in a week's time I seem to get quite illogical and irrational at the same time.'

> 'I am thirty-three years of age and have suffered from premenstrual syndrome for the best part of my adult life. The symptoms are horrible depression, muddle-headedness and deadliness. I recently took the totally unnecessary and very impulsive step of resigning from my post as a teacher of English. Of course it was just before my period that I took this drastic step. I am well qualified and have been doing this now for seven years. To all other people I appear cheerful, calm and efficient, especially when a period is not on its way.'

A specialized problem has recently arisen in the Ortho Pharmaceutical oral contraceptive plant in Puerto Rico where breast enlargement has been found among the men and menstrual disorders among the women. This has occurred in spite of the strict precautions taken in making the synthetic oestrogens. These include hermetically sealed machines, air conditioning, respirators and special protective clothing (even down to their underpants). The long-term effects of occupational exposure to oestrogens are practically unknown and there are no safety standards in force anywhere in the manufacturing of oestrogens.

How can industry cope with this unnecessary financial burden caused by menstrual problems? Fortunately most employers are supplying convenient rest rooms where a woman can relax for a few hours, take something to ease her sufferings and return to continue work for the rest of the day. The availability of flexitime, by which each worker clocks herself in and out of work at times that suit her best, is a boon to many women. They can hold a few hours in hand so that when they are at their lowest they need not go to work for that day.

Perhaps industry should tackle the problem more seriously by educating its staff, especially personnel managers and forewomen, to recognize and fully understand the problems so that women can be assigned to less skilled jobs, such as packing and stacking, during their vulnerable days rather than remaining on tasks where errors are harder to remedy later, such as soldering or filing. Some enlightened organizations arrange talks on premenstrual syndrome for their workers and managers and ensure that there are facilities for treatment locally.

Treatment centres should be available as these problems are not insoluble. Such centres should be either available in hospitals under the National Health Service, or available in centres of employment.

14

Lady's Leisure

Even when she's off duty, away from the office and housework and just relaxing, the bogey of once a month may still be with her. For among those who have led a quiet sedentary life all the week looking forward to the weekend's pleasure on the yacht, up the mountains, on the cycle, hiking, or down in the caves, which woman wants to be bothered with menstrual problems? Fortunately there's an answer for those women who are on the pill. They can be asked, when they start their initial course, 'Which day of the week would it be most convenient for you to menstruate?' and as menstruation can be expected to occur within two days of stopping the course it does not entail a very difficult calculation to decide on which day to begin. Admittedly there are some who would find it more convenient to menstruate at the weekends, when the husband can take over the household tasks and care for the children.

Sports
What about the other sporting activities in which women indulge? Those who enjoy a game of club tennis, golf or squash may well find that during the paramenstruum their performance deteriorates, for it has been found that this is the time when the arm and hand steadiness is impaired, the sharpness of vision deteriorates and there may be a slowing

of movement with the extra weight and water retention. It must not be forgotten that there are those who find the premenstrual aggression advantageous to their performance, and this includes those involved in judo and team sports. The menstrual influence on many of our top sportswomen is different, because they are chosen from those women who maintain a steady standard without fluctuations in performance. Since the mid-seventies when research by the Women's Amateur Athletics Association confirmed that one group of sportswomen, the top athletes, gave their best performance during their postmenstruum, they have arranged menstrual engineering (adjusting the time of menstruation) so that athletes at least did not have to rely on Nature's roulette.

Moller-Neilsen and Hammar from Sweden confirmed that women soccer players were more susceptible to injuries during the premenstrual and menstrual period compared with the rest of the cycle, especially among those with premenstrual symptoms of irritability, bloatedness or breast discomfort. Fewer injuries occurred among those using oral contraceptives.

The strenuous physical training schedule and weight regulation demanded of our top sportswomen all too often leads to delayed menarche, amenorrhoea, infrequent scanty menstruation, failure to ovulate or infertility. It occurs particularly in the younger age groups and those with a low body weight and low fat percentage, especially among runners, gymnasts and ballet dancers. When amenorrhoea is present, menstruation, and sometimes also ovulation, may return when training is stopped at vacations or because of injuries. Intensive physical activity can delay menarche if the activity is begun before puberty, and Frisch noted that among athletes who started training before their menarche the mean age of starting menstruation was 15.1 years, compared with athletes starting training after the menarche, who had an average menarcheal age of 12.8 years.

There is a positive correlation between athletes and the intensity of their training programme. Feicht and his colleagues showed that whereas only 6% of athletes running less than 10 miles weekly had amenorrhoea, the figure rose to 43% for those running 70 miles or more weekly. Although superficially it may seem beneficial to be without the hazards of menstruation or fear of pregnancy it is now appreciated that the lack of oestrogen can result in brittle bones in the same way as in postmenopausal women, so they become prone to stress fractures, especially of the metatarsal bones of the feet. Some studies have shown that among amenorrhaeic runners their bone mineral content was equivalent to that found in the average 52-year-old woman, which suggests that such runners need calcium and oestrogen supplementation to prevent premature osteoporosis.

Dr Ken Dyer of Adelaide has produced some interesting figures showing that over the past twenty years women's top athletic performances have improved more than men's, and suggesting that possibly within the next three or four decades women will be running and swimming as strongly as men, certainly in the longer distance races. Women have determination and aggression and are especially suited to prolonged exertion: there is a striking example of the Canadian, Cynthia Nicholas, who in the summer of 1977 set a new world record for a double crossing of the Channel in 19 hours 55 minutes, compared with the previous male record of 30 hours.

Hobbies

Women have so many hobbies that it is difficult to cover them all. There are those women who enjoy dressmaking, but will avoid cutting out a dress in an expensive material on the wrong day of the month for fear of spoiling it. Others will hesitate to spend money on flowers at that time as they find they cannot arrange them to perfection. Artists may well have difficulties and feel their inspiration is lost, and will wait until their postmenstrual peak.

Intellectual games may be affected once a month, as the partner at bridge may have discovered or the opponent at chess or Scrabble may well appreciate.

Driving Hazards

Driving is a leisure-time activity of many women. For some
it means an active participation in car rallies, while for most
it is the social journey or outing. In either case there will be
a menstrual handicap. A survey at four London hospitals
showed that half of all accident admissions of women
occurred during those vital paramenstrual days. Indeed
among those involved in an accident the menstrual influence
was equally present among the passengers, passive participants, as among the drivers, active participants. In those few
seconds which elapse between the car climbing the kerb and
before hitting a brick wall the alert passenger may brace
herself and cover her head for protection, while the passenger in her paramenstruum may be too slow or dull to take
even these elementary precautions.

Driving is a complicated task requiring the co-ordination of
many skills, which are lowered during the paramenstruum.
Complicated and rapidly changing road situations demand
instant reaction and good judgement, and if this is lowered
there may be an increase in the braking distance. The alert-
ness of hearing is decreased, so the driver may not hear
the warning hooter. The impaired sharpness of vision and
lowered ability to judge shapes and sizes means that she
loses her normal precision in parking and reversing the car.
She may be impatient of the slow driver ahead or of an
elderly person crossing the road in front of her car. She may
overtake irrationally on a blind bend or drive aggressively
round a dangerous corner. She may not respond to changing
weather conditions, failing light or alterations in the road
surfaces. She may forget to fasten her safety belt or to remember the Highway Code. Even as a pedestrian she is still
vulnerable in her paramenstruum and may cross the road
without the usual precautions, while as a mother she may
not be alert enough to guard her child from dangers on the
road. Having said all that, perhaps one should add that
women are considered by the insurance companies better
risks than men; women are only at risk during their paramenstruum, certainly not during their postmenstrual peak.

Shopping

The joys of a shopping spree may be marred during the paramenstruum. She may become an indecisive, dithering shopper who tries on all the shoes in the shop, finds they won't fit because of her swollen feet, and leaves the shop empty handed. She may buy some totally unwanted dresses, which don't fit and are the wrong colour, which she'll never wear. It is possible that her colour sense and appreciation of shape and size deteriorate during this phase of the cycle. A few women even buy unnecessary and expensive items, like furs and jewellery, merely to spite their husbands. One can't help feeling sorry for the man who wrote:

> 'I know it's the wrong day for my wife, if I come home and find the kitchen loaded with fruit, anything up to ten pounds of apples, bananas and oranges. I know she'll be in a foul temper and ask me to put the children to bed. But at other times she's the best wife in the world.'

There is the problem of women shoplifters, who are caught during the paramenstruum. While it is possible that they really are in a totally confused state and unaware of their actions, it is also possible that they are habitual shoplifters who were caught at a time when they were not sufficiently alert and did not take the usual precautions before indulging in the habit.

Entertainments

Social entertainments may not be all that successful during the paramenstruum. Cocktail parties too often require prolonged standing which isn't fun for those with water retention. As one woman put it: 'I can always recognize fellow sufferers as they also edge their way towards the walls to rest their legs.'

Other problems related to this time of the month are described:

'My problem is about ten days before a period comes. I get uncontrollable fits of depression which make me hit rock bottom. If I am with a crowd of friends I feel like I'm going to suffocate; it's a feeling that comes over me and I want to run out, and I do run out.'

'I often have to entertain for my husband. I am a good cook even if I say it myself. An excellent meal is ready but when the first guest arrives I just burst into tears. It ruins my whole evening. I've learnt to arrange my dates after my period, but then my period is bound to be late!'

Nor can the theatre bring pleasure to everyone. One sufferer from premenstrual depression recalled:

'I remember sitting in the theatre with tears rolling down my cheeks – squeezing my hands and saying to myself, "No – I mustn't, this is a comedy – everyone else is laughing." '

The problems of alcoholic intoxication are increased during the paramenstruum, so that the woman can never really let herself go without ending up in trouble. Some women can never take cannabis without suffering its worst effects, but there are those women who can take it at most times of the month and enjoy the experience. However, if they take it during the paramenstruum they may develop delusions or hallucinations.

Some women have an uncontrollable urge to gamble during the premenstruum, and the compulsion is just as bad whether it is on the horses, the dogs or in the bingo hall. One of my patient's addictions is gambling on fruit machines: on some days of the month she's just spellbound by them and can't stop. Realizing the habit, she tries to go out without any money to help remove the temptation.

Holidays

Holidays are not always as pleasurable as anticipated, and too often they can be written off as failures. There may be unexpected flight delays with the resultant food gaps. This possibility should always be borne in mind when packing, ensuring that there is an ample supply of emergency rations conveniently available. It is worth remembering that food in the plane is not served immediately after departure, nor if the plane is circling its destination for what seems hours before receiving permission to land. The hotels may have fixed hours for meals with no arrangements for mid-morning, mid-afternoon or late-night snacks.

Night travel should be avoided if at all possible, as this disturbs the day/night rhythm centre in the hypothalamus, which is close to the menstrual controlling centre. Sufferers of premenstrual syndrome are likely to have trouble with jet lag for the same reason. After a long jet flight it is worth going straight to bed regardless of the time of day at the destination, and avoiding the temptation to do some quick sightseeing or chatting with friends. A few hours' rest on arrival is well worth while in order to prevent the lethargy which results from jet lag lasting for days on end.

15

Premenstrual Syndrome Goes to Court

It was a surprising coincidence that on consecutive days, two women in different English cities appeared in court charged with murder. Both women had their charges reduced to manslaughter on the grounds of diminished responsibility caused by premenstrual syndrome. Although the circumstances of their offences were quite different, the evidence presented in each case led to the same conclusion. Each defendant was suffering from a severe case of premenstrual syndrome. Both cases had been very carefully researched and presented incontrovertible evidence of longstanding, bizarre, cyclical behaviour occurring in the premenstruum with normality of behaviour in the postmenstruum. The important point to appreciate is that these were two extreme and exceptional cases, therefore it does not mean that all sufferers of premenstrual syndrome are potential murderers, nor does it mean that all female murderers suffer from premenstrual syndrome. The International Symposium on Premenstrual, Postpartum and Menopausal Mood Disorders held at Kiawah Island in 1987 confirmed that the incidence of severe premenstrual syndrome of the type described in legal defences and expounded in the popular press was extremely small.

When a plea of premenstrual syndrome is made in the courts it is even more necessary than usual to ensure that it adheres to the strict definition. Thus there must be evidence of recurrent symptoms, or earlier episodes of a similar loss of control, confusion, amnesia or violence in previous cycles, or at monthly intervals. Women facing charges of shoplifting are often referred by their lawyers, who hope to use premenstrual syndrome as a defence. Such women are first given the definition of premenstrual syndrome and then asked, 'What did you steal in the previous two premenstruums?' This is usually enough of a shock and all too often they leave the consulting room hurriedly and try to find some other defence for their misdoings, muttering, 'But this really is my first offence.'

The necessary evidence might be found in diaries, medical records, police files, prison documents, which might give the precise dates of marital quarrels, physical violence, previous suicide attempts or slashing of the arms or legs. Indeed one woman accused of manslaughter had thirty previous convictions occurring at cycles of $29.04 + 1.47$ days, and the documents revealed that while in prison she had made attempts at drowning, strangling, escaping, slashing wrists, smashing windows and setting fire to the bed in her cell. These episodes had been meticulously recorded at the time of the event by the prison officer on duty and were found to have occurred at intervals of $29.55 + 1.45$ days. Thus the diagnosis did not rely on the woman's memory. A study of the prison records also revealed that she had been described as 'pleasant and cooperative, but at times she loses her senses and can be quite impulsive', which suggests that there was a complete absence of destructive symptoms after menstruation.

An eighteen-year-old ballet dancer accused of arson successfully pleaded premenstrual syndrome as a mitigating factor and was released on probation. She had an excellent school report and her behaviour was exemplary until menstruation started, when she appeared to change in character and since then had episodes of unusual and unexplained behaviour. One day she suddenly went into her bedroom and shaved off her blonde hair and eyebrows; on another occasion she ran away from home and was later returned by police having been found drunk and disorderly; once she burnt the bedroom curtains; another time she overdosed herself with pain relievers and alcohol and was admitted to hospital overnight; finally she set fire to her father's house and was admitted to prison. While in prison she attempted to set fire to the bed in her cell, and on another occasion she attempted strangling by tying one end of her sheet around her neck and the other end to the top of the window. It was her father who noticed from his diaries that these problems with his daughter occurred about once a month. He was advised to produce proof of the precise dates on which the many curious happenings occurred. There followed a search of the doctor's and hospital's files, dates of insurance claims for the burnt curtains, the cheque date on which he bought his daughter a new wig, and the precise dates on which she misbehaved while in prison. Again, the many occurrences were shown to be coming in regular monthly cycles. She received progesterone treatment and is now a successful executive.

A similar story can be told of an unemployed girl who harassed the police with unnecessary emergency phone calls. Earlier she had been in reform school for such phone calls, but on release the emergency phone calls persisted and disrupted normal police work. She was imprisoned. Her father again was the one who noticed that the problems arose each month and drew the lawyer's attention to the coincidences. In her case it represented a cry for help, akin to the other woman whose cry for attention might be a suicide attempt or slashed arms or legs. She too responded to progesterone and was released on probation. However, on her return to civilian life progesterone was not restarted and she again made unnecessary police phone calls. This time, no mercy was shown. She served her two-year sentence. That was six years ago; on progesterone treatment her life has changed and she now works with the disabled, is happily married and has one son.

In 1977 a 46-year-old part-time social worker faced a charge of shoplifting. In evidence she produced a diary showing the days of confusion each month, when she refused to leave the house, and she arranged her days at work accordingly.

Her husband had recognized these cyclical occasions of confusion and described how she would return home from shopping with dog food, although they kept no animals, or a child's ski outfit although their own children were now adult. Together with his wife they would mark in the diary the days on which trouble might occur. All was well until a member of staff caught 'flu and the social worker agreed to alter her working days. The case was dismissed. She has since received progesterone treatment and been free from these lapses of concentration and confusion.

These represent genuine cases of criminal behaviour resulting from a hormonal disease and responding to treatment. These women should rightly be freed for they cannot be held responsible for their sudden unexpected loss of control. However, the genuine cases are few and far between. A far bigger problem has now arisen and it is our duty to ensure that premenstrual syndrome is not made a universal defence. Already cases have occurred in Britain where this has been tried. A woman on her first charge of shoplifting cannot make a claim of premenstrual syndrome without evidence that this is a recurrent offence. The mere coincidence of two car crashes, or two speeding offences, occurring in the premenstruum is insufficient evidence of premenstrual syndrome. The public have a right to be protected by the knowledge that the defendant is receiving progesterone treatment and is unlikely to be a further danger to the public. At a recent appeal trial in Britain premenstrual syndrome as a defence in a case of murder was rejected, although it still stands as 'a factor causing diminished responsibility' in capital charges and as 'a mitigating factor' in lesser charges.

For the correct diagnosis of premenstrual syndrome, the precise dates of menstruation and of the alleged crime are a prerequisite. Yet a clerk in a travel agency, accused of stealing travellers' cheques worth £500 from her employer at some unknown date between August 1980 and April 1981, pleaded premenstrual syndrome. Not surprisingly the plea failed and a jail sentence was imposed.

Offences committed by sufferers of premenstrual syndrome have certain characteristics which may be easily recognized.

- 1 The woman acts alone without an accomplice.
- 2 The offence is not premeditated, and usually comes as a surprise to anyone she was with shortly before the event.
- 3 The action is without apparent motive, such as setting fire to an unknown person's property.
- 4 There may be no attempt to escape detection. A woman randomly throwing a brick at a shop window may herself telephone the police and await her arrest.
- 5 The action may be a *cri de coeur*, as with the hoaxer who repeatedly makes emergency 999 calls. This is similar to a parasuicide.

Among the more frequent symptoms of premenstrual syndrome, which may result in criminal charges, are a sudden and momentary surge of uncontrollable emotions resulting in violence, confusion or amnesia, alcoholism, nymphomania and attention-seeking episodes which represent cries for help. These cover a full range of criminal offences, such as actual violence, damage to property, theft and disorderly behaviour.

Sufferers of premenstrual syndrome characteristically have painfree menstruation. The shoplifter who claimed her period pains were so severe that she was under the influence of pain-relieving drugs at the time of her offence was suffering from spasmodic dysmenorrhoea, and not from premenstrual syndrome.

A full medical history will reveal many features which confirm or refute the diagnosis. The onset of premenstrual syndrome, and the occasions of increased severity, always occur at times of hormonal upheaval, as at puberty, or after using the pill, after a spell of amenorrhoea, pregnancy or sterilization. These are the women who have side effects on the oral contraceptive pill, and their pregnancies may be complicated by pre-eclampsia or postnatal depression. During the premenstruum they have difficulty in tolerating long intervals without food and they easily become intoxicated by alcohol in the premenstruum.

A 32-year-old Essex housewife was accused of infanticide, having drowned her second daughter and then overdosed herself. She started menstruating in the intensive care unit and mention of premenstrual syndrome was noted in her previous medical records. Some years earlier she had developed migraine and hypertension on the pill, for which she had been admitted to the London Hospital for observation. Her first pregnancy was complicated by pre-eclampsia and after her second she developed postnatal depression requiring a psychiatric domicillary visit. The incident had occurred at about 5.30 p.m.; she had no food since her 8.30 a.m. breakfast. The court accepted the several diagnostic pointers of premenstrual syndrome and she was released on probation with a treatment order.

Increased libido may be a problem among young women suffering from premenstrual syndrome. All too often it is this nymphomanic urge in adolescents which is responsible for young girls running away from home, or custody, only to be found wandering in the park or following the boys. These girls can be helped, and their criminal career abruptly ended with hormone therapy.

Some women are needlessly incarcerated due to premenstrual syndrome. They are deserving of our sympathy, and justice will not be served until all true sufferers of premenstrual syndrome are properly diagnosed and treated. The road to rehabilitation after a prison sentence is long and hard. Feminine interests will be best served by increasing our diagnostic capacity, enabling us to distinguish the few genuine sufferers from the many malingerers who are trying to jump on the bandwagon and whose claims of premenstrual syndrome can never be substantiated.*

* Further information on this subject is contained in my book *Premenstrual Syndrome Goes to Court*, published by Peter Andrew Publishing Company, Droitwich, Worcestershire (1990).

The Hormonal Control

Some scientists believe that the body is governed by bio-rhythms, which include a physical rhythm of 23 days, a sensitivity or emotional rhythm of 28 days and an intellectual rhythm of 33 days. These body cycles are not affected by life's events and repeat themselves so unchangingly that they can be worked out for any individual by anyone who can count, or by computer, provided only that the hour and date of birth are known. Under no circumstances should the menstrual cycle be associated with biorhythms, for it is completely different. No matter how precisely you can pin-point the hour and date of birth, this will not enable you or anyone else to work out when the menstrual cycle will begin, what its length will be or anything at all about its pattern of ovulation and menstruation.

The menstrual cycle does not begin at birth. It is interrupted by pregnancy and breast feeding and is altered by life's events such as illnesses, examinations, bereavement, happy events, sad events and changes in environment. Further-more, menstrual patterns show endless variations in duration of flow, quantity of blood lost, as well as the length of cycle.

When teaching about the menstrual cycle it is easiest if one considers only a 28-day cycle. It makes for simplicity and is easier when discussing the various changes, such as ovu-lation on the fourteenth day. But we must not lose sight of the fact that women are all individuals and do not fit naturally into such neat pigeon-holes. Sometimes one is asked, 'What is the right length of the menstrual cycle?' They might as well ask, 'What is the right height for a woman?' All individuals are different: one meets many healthy normal women who menstruate about every 21 days, as well as those at the other extreme who only menstruate on average every 36 days. Both are quite normal with fully effective reproductive systems. The cycle of 28 days is only the average of all women all over the world.

It is said that Dr Pinkus, the father of the pill, decided over a cup of tea with the British endocrinologist, Peter Bishop, that 28 days would be a convenient time interval to allow withdrawal bleeding to occur in women on the pill. So it is that today there are millions of women with man-made cycles of 28 days. But they could just as easily have decided on 24 or 30 days.

Chiazze and his colleagues found that only 62% of women aged 15–19 years had a menstrual cycle between 25 and 31 days, but the proportion of women gradually increased with age so that between 35 and 39 years there were 86% with an almost conventional cycle. When women are asked the length of their cycle the frequent reply is, 'Oh, I'm always late,' meaning it is more than 28 days, or, 'I'm quite regular,' meaning 'I never have to get worried because I'm never over 28 days.' Incidentally, when counting the days of a cycle it should be counted from the first day of menstruation until the first day of the next menstruation. Confusion sometimes occurs because women count from the end of one period until the beginning of the next – they only count the days they are not bleeding.

The duration in the time of menstrual flow varies too from cycle to cycle and from individual to individual. It may be for as short as two days or go on as long as eight days, and still the doctors would consider it normal and know that these women would be able to have children if this was their desire. The quantity of the menstrual flow, or blood loss, is also variable, and as no two people are likely to see another person's flow there is bound to be considerable exaggeration in both directions. Some women will even say, 'I had a really good period,' which can be interpreted as meaning the loss was bright red. Many women object to the scanty dark red, brown or black loss which sometimes comes with the pill. It is as well to realize that menstrual bleeding comes from the minute blood vessels of the lining of the womb, and not from any big blood vessels, so that if bleeding continued for a very long time it might cause anaemia, but one can never actually bleed to death as one could from a wound in a limb.

The type of flow is also different in different women. Some start with a heavy loss, which continues for a few days and then stops abruptly. Others start more gradually, with one or two days of scanty loss before the full flow, and then end either abruptly or gradually over a few days. All these types are normal, but the symptoms of premenstrual syndrome do not end until the full menstrual flow, so that some women may have problems during the first few days of menstruation.

The Menstrual Controlling Centre

In the opening chapter the menstrual cycle was broken down into seven four-day phases of hormone activity. Each hormone change is carefully monitored by the control centre, often referred to as the 'menstrual clock', which is not situated in the womb where the action takes place, but at a distance from it low in the brain, in the part known as the 'hypothalamus', where it can receive impulses or messages from the brain (Fig. 20). The hypothalamus is itself the control centre of many other functions, among them being the centre for the control of water balance, of appetite, of weight, of mood, and of day/night rhythm, so that if any one of these is upset it will tend to affect the others. The diagram in Fig. 21 shows the proximity of these centres, which explains why, when the menstrual cycle is disturbed, as it is by taking the pill, this can upset the weight, the water balance and the mood centre, causing in turn a gain in weight, water retention and depression. In a similar way, if the appetite is drastically curtailed, as in anorexia nervosa, the menstrual cycle

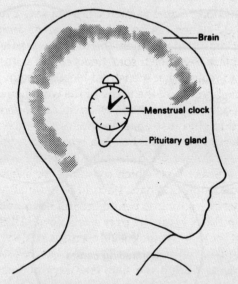

It is at the base of the brain in the Hypothalamus, above
the Pituitary gland.

Fig. 20 Position of the menstrual clock

will be stopped and depression will develop. Again, depressive illnesses are likely to cause an alteration in menstruation,
resulting in either excessive bleeding, as in the 'weeping
womb', or menstruation ceasing. It can also cause alterations
in weight, either a gain or a loss.

The diurnal controlling centre, which is concerned with
sleep rhythm, is also situated in the hypothalamus close to
the menstrual clock. Those with a sensitive menstrual clock
are likely to be easily upset by night-shift working and have
marked jet lag after long flights.

Menstrual Clock

The menstrual clock, being the control centre of the
menstrual cycle, is responsible for the smooth and effective
operation of the woman's marvellous reproductive system.

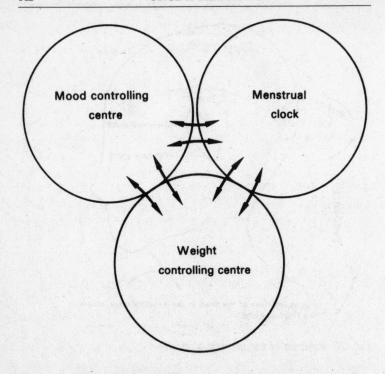

Fig. 21 Diagram of controlling centres in the hypothalamus

Situated in the hypothalamus, it has two hormones which it uses for this purpose. Hormones are chemicals with their own individual structure and designed to act on a particular target organ. They are chemical messengers travelling in the bloodstream. These two hormones have very grand-sounding names, 'follicle stimulating hormone releasing hormone' (FSHRH) and 'luteinizing hormone releasing hormone' (LHRH). Their target is the pituitary gland situated next to the hypothalamus at the base of the brain. The effect of these two releasing hormones from the hypothalamus is to stimulate the pituitary gland to produce two other menstrual hormones, *follicle stimulating hormone* (FSH) and *luteinizing hormone* (LH), boosting the hormone output (Fig. 22).

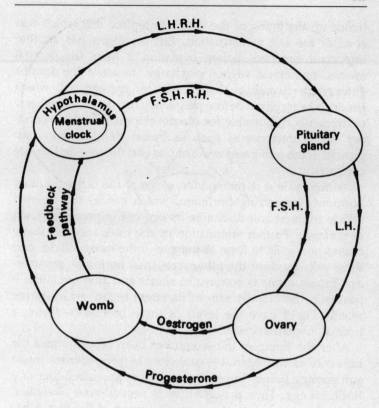

L.H.R.H.

F.S.H.R.H.

Hypothalamus
Menstrual
clock

Pituitary
gland

Feedback
pathway

F.S.H.

L.H.

Womb

Oestrogen

Ovary

Progesterone

Fig. 22 Menstrual hormonal pathways

The pituitary gland sends out a variety of different hormones which control, among other things, growth, pigmentation, lactation, thyroid, adrenal and insulin output. In short it has a finger in every pie. But what concerns us now are the two pituitary hormones, follicle stimulating hormone and luteinizing hormone, which act on the ovary. The follicle stimulating hormone acts on the ovaries by stimulating the formation of follicles, or tiny microscopic rings of cells within which is an immature ovum, or egg cell. As the follicles develop, specialized cells produce *oestrogen*, yet another hormone, which is released into the bloodstream. Oestrogen builds up the lining of the womb to replace that which was shed at the last menstruation. But oestrogen has another important function. Before ovulation it thins the cervical mucus, or natural vaginal discharge, to assist the sperms entering the womb in their search for the egg cell, which needs to be fertilized before pregnancy can occur. At puberty oestrogen is responsible for the development of the secondary sex characteristics, such as breast development, hair growth in the pubic area and armpits and the rounded female contours.

At mid-cycle it is the sudden surge of the other pituitary hormone, luteinizing hormone, which causes the ripened follicle to burst and discharge its egg cell, a process known as *ovulation*. Further stimulation by the luteinizing hormone causes new cells to form at the site of the burst follicle, and these cells produce the other menstrual hormone, *progesterone*. Progesterone is secreted in spurts and after ovulation it passes in the bloodstream to its target organ, which is the womb. Fig. 1 gave the levels of these hormones during a normal menstrual cycle.

After the lining of the womb has been rebuilt under the influence of oestrogen it is converted by progesterone into a soft spongy lining, hopefully ready for the embedding of a fertilized egg. Thus progesterone is needed after ovulation, when the initial repair work on the lining of the womb has already taken place. Progesterone is also responsible for making the fallopian tubes contract more forcefully, but less frequently, so that the egg cell may be swept along to the womb. Progesterone also changes the vaginal discharge from the thin watery fluid in which sperm could move freely into a thick, sticky mucus, thus preventing further sperm entering the womb. The presence of progesterone raises the body temperature, again in preparation for a possible pregnancy.

Nature has devised a magnificent machine in our reproductive system, complete with a highly efficient intercommunication system between the hypothalamus, pituitary, ovary and womb which is called the 'feedback pathway'. This ensures that the higher centres are kept fully informed of the progress in the ovaries and the womb (Fig. 22) and can alter the level of hormones according to the information received. For instance should conception occur the hormonal output is altered within hours. Another important control is *prolactin*, a hormone produced by the anterior pituitary gland which regulates the progesterone feedback mechanism so that if too much prolactin is produced the progesterone feedback pathway is interrupted.

Ovulation

Most women recognize when ovulation occurs as there may be a slight sensation of discomfort for about an hour in one side of the lower abdomen, and at the same time they may notice that their normal vaginal discharge changes from a thin fluid to a thick, sticky mucus. Some women have a migraine at that time or a tendency to irritability, while for the more unfortunate women it may herald the onset of premenstrual syndrome. Sometimes when the migraine or irritability at ovulation is severe women have difficulty in becoming pregnant because they avoid having intercourse on the very days that they are most likely to conceive.

If a woman carefully records her temperature for two minutes every morning before getting out of bed it may be possible to decide whether or not she is ovulating and also whether she has sufficient progesterone. In Fig. 23 a few temperature charts are shown. Teresa is normal; ovulation occurred as shown by the sudden dip and subsequent raised temperature until the start of menstruation. Ursula's chart is very steady, and all on the same level with no evidence of ovulation; it is known as an 'anovular chart'. Victoria's chart does show ovulation, and a rise of temperature, but this rise is not maintained suggesting that she has insufficient progesterone and a short luteal phase. It must be appreciated that temperature charts are not always reliable; ovulation can occur even with a chart like Ursula's.

The exact time of ovulation can be determined in several ways; by the change from a thin discharge to thick, sticky

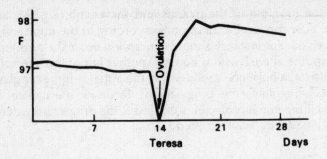

Teresa   Days

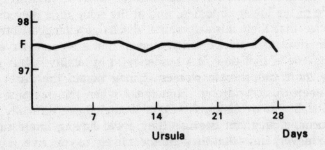

Ursula   Days

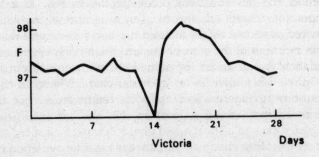

Victoria   Days

Fig. 23 Temperature charts taken through the menstrual cycle

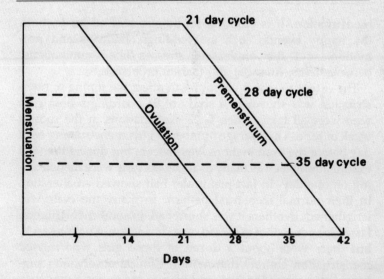

Fig. 24 Timing of ovulation with different lengths of cycles

mucus, a daily temperature chart, tests showing the time of the peak of luteinizing hormone in the blood, and direct inspection of the ovary either at the time of an abdominal operation or by laparoscopy, in which a minute periscope is inserted through the abdominal wall; but the most reliable method is by serial ultrasound scans of the ovaries. Ovulation occurs 12–14 days before the onset of menstruation, so it is only correct to talk about ovulation at mid-cycle in one whose cycle averages 28 days, but in those who have a longer cycle ovulation will be occurring after mid-cycle as shown in Fig. 24. In women with a 35-day cycle ovulation is likely to occur about day 21, whereas in those with a short cycle of 21 days it is more likely to occur about day 10.

Emotional Upset of Menstruation
The menstrual clock is a very delicate mechanism which requires an exact hormone balance to ensure a trouble-free

menstruation. It is easily upset by stress of all kinds, both
the happy events, such as weddings, holidays and promotion, and the unpleasant stresses like examinations,
bereavements, financial and marital problems.

The extent to which emotion can affect the timing of menstruation was shown in a study of 91 boarding-school girls
who were all taking their GCE examinations in the second
week of June. The average number of girls menstruating each
day before the examinations was sixteen, but during the vital
examination week as many as thirty-six girls were menstruating on one day. In fact just under half showed an alteration
in their normal menstrual pattern. In many the cycle was
lengthened, in others it was shortened, in some menstruation
lasted longer so that it spread over during examination week,
but there were about a dozen of those girls who missed
menstruation entirely that month. Clinical observation suggests that each individual's reaction to stress has a tendency
to be the same throughout their menstruating years, so that
the girls who missed the menstruation at the time of examinations might also stop suddenly in later life if they were
molested or their homes burnt down. The others, who
reacted with prolonged menstrual loss, might similarly
expect to react in the same way under severe stress.

One letter-writer asked:

> 'Since my husband was killed in a sailing accident last year
> my periods have been very irregular and much heavier. I
> have now got over the loss, have got a new job and only
> get depressed before a period. Is this anything to worry
> about?'

No, a horrible shock like that is bound to be felt by the
hypothalamus, which in turn will temporarily upset the
normal menstrual pattern. As she appears to be adjusting
her life to the tragedy it is likely that gradually her menstruation will return to its old pattern.

Menstrual Synchrony

Another point to be considered in relation to the timing of menstruation is what is called *menstrual synchrony*, which is when a number of women's menstruations occur together. This happens among women who live closely together in closed communities, like communes, prisons, convents, college campuses and school dormitories; and especially if they share common emotional experiences, such as examinations and end-of-term excitement, their menstruation gradually becomes synchronized. This in turn raises fresh problems for it also means that if more than one woman is suffering from premenstrual tension trouble is inevitable. Indeed, it may be necessary to move women prisoners from one cell to another before such synchronization occurs. Menstrual synchrony is frequently noticed with mothers and daughters. If a daughter is brought to the doctor by her mother and is unable to remember the date of her last menstruation, the chances are that the mother will reply and then add, 'Our dates always come together.' Similarly, menstruation tends to coincide among lesbians. The mechanism of this synchronization is not clear, but it has been suggested that it may be related to sensitivity to body odours or pheromones.

The potency of these menstrual hormones is almost unbelievable. The powder a woman uses to cover the tip of her nose weighs many times more than the total amount of female hormones to be found in her bloodstream. Yet they cause the sex organs and breasts to grow to mature size, and they bring about changes in bone structure and fat distribution which mould her figure into feminine contours and bring her to the peak of womanhood and motherhood.

Sex Hormone Binding Globulin

Hormones are chemical messengers made in one organ and having their action on some other tissue. Sex hormones can be attached, or bound, in the blood to a minute protein molecule called 'globulin'. The capacity of this sex hormone binding globulin to bind to dihydrotestosterone is measured in the SHBG estimation, mentioned on page 27. Just where this fits into the jigsaw of premenstrual syndrome is at present unknown. Why is the SHBG low in premenstrual syndrome? Why does the low SHBG rise when progesterone is administered to sufferers of premenstrual syndrome? Again, why does the SHBG fall when progestogens are administered? This only emphasizes the many riddles which are still awaiting solutions in order to further our understanding of premenstrual syndrome.

Hormone Receptors

When a hormone has travelled in the blood to the tissue where its action is required, it is transported to the cell nucleus by means of a *hormone receptor*. Hormone receptors are situated within the tissue cells and key on to a single molecule of their special hormone and convey it through the cell substance and the nuclear wall into the nucleus, where the hormone is converted and used. Hormone receptors are very specific, and will only transport the special hormone for which they are made, be it thyroid, cortisone, oestrogen or progesterone. Progesterone receptors are present in the lining of the womb where their presence is understandable, but their distribution in other parts of the body is of special interest for they represent tissues which utilize progesterone in the luteal phases, although the precise purpose of progesterone within these cells is not yet fully known. Progesterone receptors are widespread in the body. The largest concentration is found in the limbic area of the mid-brain, a part of the brain that animal biologists refer to as the 'area of rage and violence'. It seems possible that it is an insufficiency of progesterone receptors in the mid-brain which is responsible for premenstrual tension. Progesterone receptors are also found in the nasopharangeal passages and lungs, eyes, breast and liver. Consideration of other premenstrual symptoms suggests that they occur in just those areas: namely the nasopharangeal passages and lungs (responsible for rhinitis, sinusitis, laryngitis and asthma); the eyes (responsible for conjunctivitis, styes, uveitis and glaucoma); and the breasts (responsible for mastitis). This widespread distribution of progesterone receptors in target cells explains the numerous different symptoms of premenstrual syndrome.

When progesterone is taken by mouth it passes via the portal system to the liver, the site of numerous progesterone receptors, where it is broken down and converted into other substances, different from the metabolic substances resulting from the breakdown of progesterone in other tissues. With oral progesterone the concentration of hormone reaching the systemic blood is considerably lower. There are no hormone receptors for the man-made progestogen drugs, although they may sometimes force themselves into progesterone receptors or testosterone receptors, but they do not do this equally well in all the progesterone receptor sites in the body.

With increased knowledge has come the realization that hormones do not have a single action, but act on many systems. One has only to think of the widespread effects of an excess of thyroid or a deficiency of insulin in diabetes. Thus, in addition to the action of oestrogen on the reproductive system, it is also involved in cholesterol balance, bone metabolism, blood circulation and maintaining elasticity of the skin.

Progesterone

Irene Elias in the *Female Animal* reminds us that progesterone is the oldest steroid on the evolutionary scale, being some five hundred million years old, and that progesterone is present in all vertebrates, including frogs, snakes, birds and fishes. It will readily be appreciated that not all vertebrates menstruate nor do they all require progesterone for reproduction, but in the lower vertebrates progesterone is involved in glucose metabolism and the development of intelligence. The role of progesterone in the enhancement of intelligence has been demonstrated in my surveys of 1968 and 1976 when 32% of children, whose mothers received progesterone during pregnancy, went on to university compared with 6%

of controls (who were the next born children in the labour ward register); 6% is also the national average. Progesterone is also present in the adrenals in men, women and children and is converted into other steroid hormones, such as cortisone, oestrogen and testosterone.

Progesterone Receptors

The study of the characteristics of progesterone receptors has relied on animal studies as there have been no volunteers for brain biopsies from normal women or from premenstrual syndrome sufferers. However, we have learnt from molecular biologists that, since progesterone is a steroid, its molecules can pass through the cell wall into the substance of the cell, but that once there the molecules need to combine with progesterone receptors to form a 'hormone receptor complex' in order to be transported into the nucleus and DNA, where it is broken down and used.

Blaustein has demonstrated the ability of progesterone receptors to accept an initial dose of progesterone, but subsequent doses need to be some forty times the original dose before they can form a hormone receptor complex. No explanation has yet been given for this surprising progesterone receptor requirement. However, it is known that during pregnancy the progesterone blood level rises some forty times above the peak level found in the luteal phase of the menstrual cycle (Fig 25). This massive increase in progesterone is produced by the placenta within the womb and is essentially for the benefit of the foetus. Nevertheless, it is known that women with premenstrual syndrome are entirely free from their premenstrual symptoms during the latter half of pregnancy, and indeed many blossom at this time, which would seem to indicate that they are sharing with the foetus this massive increase in progesterone production. Could it be that there is a central control system which, whilst ensuring a sufficiency for the developing foetus, controls the distribution of any surplus to the mother? If this control system failed to return to a normal prepregnancy state, it might account for the resurgence of premenstrual symptoms or the development of postnatal depression immediately after the delivery of the placenta. It might also explain why premenstrual syndrome so frequently starts or increases in severity after a pregnancy, as the possible result of insufficient progesterone to stimulate the progesterone receptors. It would also explain the failure of low-dose progesterone used in double blind trials, which have never shown the beneficial effect of high-dose progesterone used by the clinician. There is no evidence of any such high requirement of oestrogen molecules by oestrogen receptors, and so the doses of oestrogen used in hormone replacement therapy are physiological, usually only one or two milligrams.

Another important characteristic of progesterone receptors demonstrated by Nock is that they cannot convey molecules of progesterone to the nucleus of cells in the presence of adrenalin.

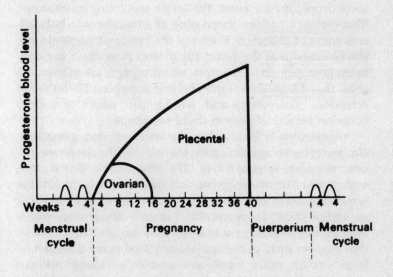

Fig. 25 Levels of progesterone during the menstrual cycle and pregnancy

Blood Sugar Level

Progesterone also plays a part in the regulation of the blood sugar (or blood glucose) level. To ensure that the blood sugar always remains within the optimum level there are two regulating mechanisms, an upper and a lower. These prevent the blood sugar level becoming too high (hyperglycaemic), or too low (hypoglycaemic), when there is a danger of loss of consciousness or death (Fig. 26). The blood sugar is maintained by eating carbohydrates, the energy-giving foods, which cover the starches (flour, potatoes, oats, rye and rice) and the sugars. The effect of eating sugars is to cause a rapid rise and rapid drop in the blood sugar level, whereas ingestion of starches brings a more sustained rise and slower fall. If a large quantity of carbohydrate is eaten at one meal the upper regulating mechanism is brought into play, there is a surge of insulin and a valve opens, releasing the extra sugar into the urine (renal threshold). On the other hand if there is a long interval without food and the blood sugar level drops, it may reach the lower regulating mechanism. This causes a sudden outpouring of adrenalin which mobilizes some of the sugar stored in the cells and passes it into the blood so that the blood sugar level is again at the optimum level (Fig. 26). However, when sugar is taken from the cells, they fill up with water and this is responsible for water retention, bloatedness and weight gain which is such a common feature of premenstrual syndrome.

Progesterone is involved in the lower regulating mechanism and if before menstruation there is insufficient progesterone, the level is raised (Fig. 27). This means that women with premenstrual syndrome will tend to reach the level at which the lower regulating mechanism comes into action at an earlier stage. In practice it is usually about three hours after ingestion of starchy food, so they are advised to ensure that they eat small portions of starchy food every three hours. Men, on the other hand, can usually go longer without replenishment as their lower regulating mechanism is set at a different level.

Adrenalin is the hormone which mobilizes the body's

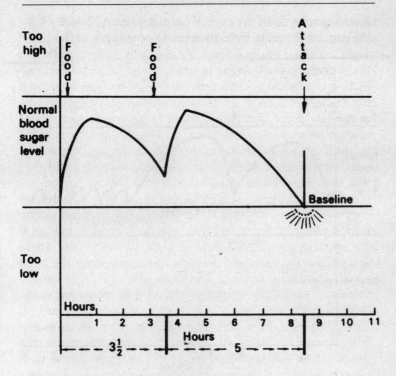

Fig. 26 Effect of food on blood sugar levels

defences against 'fright, fight and flight', and this sudden outpouring of adrenalin may be enough to trigger off a sudden fit of irritability, migraine, panic or epilepsy. In others it may cause them to feel weak, shivery, faint or bring on palpitations. On the other hand there are also those fortunate individuals who can manage long fasts, as they are unaware when their blood sugar baseline has been reached, and they get renewed energy from their own sugar stores.

These attacks brought on by fasting are sometimes erroneously called 'hypoglycaemic attacks', but doctors don't like that word as hypoglycaemia is reserved for those whose blood sugar stays below the baseline and below the normal blood sugar level. In the case of normal women Nature's fail-safe control prevents hypoglycaemia occurring.

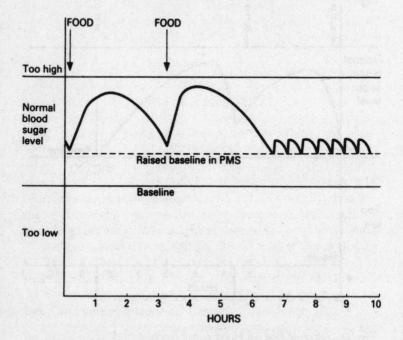

Fig. 27 *Effect of food on blood sugar levels in women with premenstrual syndrome*

17

What Goes Wrong?

The cause of premenstrual syndrome is a subject most research workers avoid. Even medical journals prefer publishing failed treatment trials rather than discussing what goes wrong to cause premenstrual syndrome. Any theory into its cause must embrace all the known facts, such as:

- 1 It only occurs in women during the reproductive years.
- 2 Symptoms are present in the premenstruum and absent in the postmenstruum.
- 3 Symptoms are absent during the second half of pregnancy, but severe attacks occur after delivery.
- 4 Symptoms start at puberty, after a pregnancy, after a spell of amenorrhoea, after stopping the pill, after sterilization and after hysterectomy and/or oophorectomy. These are all times when the menstrual controlling centre in the brain has been upset.
- 5 Premenstrual syndrome can occur in both ovular and anovular cycles and can be present in the year or two before menstruation starts and after it ends.
- 6 The 150 symptoms which may occur in premenstrual syndrome can also occur in men, children and postmenopausal women. There are more somatic than psychological symptoms.
- 7 Women with premenstrual syndrome have difficulty

in tolerating long intervals without food and are liable to binges, especially for sweet foods.

- 8 Symptoms increase at times of stress and when there has been a long interval without food.

- 9 There is a good response to systemic progesterone if given in high doses, although double blind controlled trials of low-dose progesterone in premenstrual syndrome suggest progesterone is no better than a placebo.

- 10 Studies have shown that premenstrual syndrome is not related to blood levels of progesterone, oestrogen, FSH, LH, aldosterone, prolactin or serotonin.

All these facts need to be covered in any satisfactory explanation of the cause of premenstrual syndrome.

Progesterone Receptors are the Key

Recent work in molecular biochemistry has revealed the importance of progesterone receptors in the body's utilization of the circulating progesterone, and an understanding of the unique characteristics of progesterone receptors and glucocorticoid receptors (see pages 150–3) has provided an explanation for all the facts enumerated above. It is suggested that progesterone receptors are the missing link in our understanding of premenstrual syndrome: either there are insufficient progesterone receptors to transport the molecules of progesterone into the nucleus, or the ability of the receptors is inhibited by adrenalin or some unknown factor.

Spasmodic Dysmenorrhoea

It has already been mentioned that spasmodic dysmenorrhoea is the opposite to premenstrual syndrome and there are several factors which suggest that oestrogen deficiency lies at the cause of these period pains. For instance:

- 1 It does not start with the first menstruation, but only when ovulation occurs.
- 2 It is relieved by a full-term pregnancy.
- 3 If a pregnancy does not intervene, a gradual reduction in pain after the age of 25 years is usual.
- 4 The pain is relieved by the pill or oestrogen administration.
- 5 The sufferers tend to be immature, with poor breast development and sparse hair in their armpits.
- 6 It is frequently accompanied by acne.

At puberty, oestrogen is responsible for the development of the secondary sex characteristics. It is responsible for the pubertal breast development, for the development of hair in the armpits and lower abdomen, for the development and enlargement of the womb, and more especially for developing the muscles of the womb and ensuring that it has a good blood supply. Oestrogen decreases the production of grease in the skin and so prevents acne. An important action of oestrogen is the reduction of prostaglandin released by the lining cells of the womb (endometrium). Prostaglandin is a chemical released by cells when they are damaged. Many different types of prostaglandins have been isolated. The particular prostaglandins released by endometrial cells are known as F2 alpha, and it has been shown that the level of prostaglandin F2 alpha in the blood is raised in women with spasmodic dysmenorrhoea.

If ovular menstruation occurs before the womb is fully developed, the door to the womb is not supple enough to open easily for the flow of menstrual blood. It is rather like trying to blow up a balloon for the first time, which is very difficult, but if it has once been fully inflated then on the next occasion it is easy to inflate. If the womb is gradually stretched during the nine months of pregnancy then subsequently the door will open up at menstruation without pain. Or if the muscles of the womb are gradually increased by the prolonged action of oestrogen the painful periods are gradually eased during the mid-twenties.

Two Hormonal Types

Thus it would seem that the two common period problems, premenstrual syndrome and spasmodic dysmenorrhoea, are related to a deficiency in the levels of the two menstrual hormones, progesterone and oestrogen respectively. Fig. 28 shows a diagram of the effect of these two hormone levels on an individual. A marked progesterone deficiency will cause severe premenstrual syndrome, while a mild deficiency will cause only mild premenstrual syndrome. On the other hand a moderately low oestrogen level will only cause mild spasmodic dysmenorrhoea, but a severe oestrogen deficiency will cause severe period pains. In between these two are those fortunate women who do not experience any problems with menstruation. Although women may move slightly up and down this scale during the course of their lives, the movement will tend to stay within the limits of the same group, unless either progesterone or oestrogen is given or a

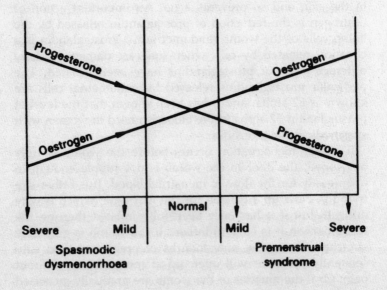

Fig. 28 Arbitrary levels of progesterone and oestrogen

pregnancy occurs. These two groups of women tend to have other common characteristics.

Progesterone Deficient Group

Women in the premenstrual syndrome group will tend to be fertile, but their pregnancies may be followed by postnatal depression, and they are more prone to depressive illnesses and high blood pressure during their life span. Among those who become pregnant one in every five will be likely to have pre-eclamptic toxaemia, with a marked gain in weight and high blood pressure during pregnancy, while the others will blossom in pregnancy being free from their usual premenstrual migraine, asthma and depression and will later look back on the last months of pregnancy as the healthiest days of their life. These women, if given oestrogen, will tend to get side effects as they already have a high level of this hormone. They will be prone to the minor side effects of nausea, gain in weight, headaches and depression, but will also risk the more serious ones like thrombosis. The pill contains oestrogen, together with a synthetic progestogen, and as already mentioned progestogens lower the normal progesterone level in the blood, so making their existing progesterone deficiency worse.

Oestrogen Deficient Group

On the other hand, the woman with spasmodic dysmenorrhoea will grow out of her period pains, either following pregnancy or during the mid-twenties, and thereafter will have trouble-free menstruation. These are the women who feel positively better on the pill, even preferring the ones with the relatively higher dose of oestrogen, as these boost their low oestrogen levels. However, at the menopause their already low oestrogen levels are not helped by the declining oestrogen output from the ovaries, so these women are likely to develop their menopausal symptoms early, even before menstruation has stopped, and unless they are given replacement treatment during the menopausal years they are likely to be the ones who suffer most from the ending of their childbearing years.

As with other hormonal disorders it is not surprising to find that there is a marked family tendency with daughters, sisters and mother belonging to the same menstrual hormonal group, either progesterone deficient or oestrogen deficient.

Studies of identical twins have shown that if one suffers from premenstrual syndrome then the other will also, whereas in unidentical twins the incidence of premenstrual syndrome is the same as that found among sisters. Similarly, adopted daughters are likely to take the pattern of their natural mother in respect of either premenstrual syndrome or spasmodic dysmenorrhoea, and not the pattern of their adopted mother.

Missed Periods

> 'Married hopes and unmarried fear
> Are the common cause of amenorrhoea.'

Amenorrhoea is the absence of periods, and the above quoted nurses' jingle is a reminder that the commonest cause of a missed menstruation is pregnancy. Often, if the woman is single, it is more likely to be a delayed period, since she normally may have a long cycle of perhaps 33–36 days, and because she has not kept a record of her cycles and has run a risk during the month she is fearful, on every day after the 28th day, that she might be pregnant. Unfortunately, as yet, the routine pregnancy test cannot be used reliably until two weeks after the missed period, or 42 days since the last period, and this is an awful long time to wait. However, there would usually be the tell-tale signs of an early pregnancy such as morning sickness, getting up to pass water at night and painful enlarging breasts.

An HCG blood test can recognize a pregnancy within

seven days of conception, which is even before the missed period. HCG stands for 'human chorionic gonadotrophin' which is one of the special pregnancy hormones released immediately after conception. Similarly, serial ultrasound scans of the ovaries will detect an early pregnancy within days of embedding in the womb. However both these are expensive methods and not universally available. There used to be a hormonal pregnancy test in which oestrogen and progestogen tablets were taken and, if the woman was not pregnant, vaginal bleeding would occur within 48 hours. This test has now been stopped due to the ever-present risk that, should the woman be pregnant, the test might cause foetal abnormalities.

Missed periods may occur quite normally at puberty, during the first three years after the onset of menstruation, during breast feeding and again at the menopause. In the last case, menstruation has often started to get shorter and the loss lighter before a period is actually missed.

To find the other causes of missed menstruation one must return to the hormonal controlling system, for any upset to the hormonal pathway may disturb the normal rhythm of menstruation. Stress is perhaps the commonest cause:

A friend, WINIFRED, with two children, had been visiting us but when she returned to her home she found a fire engine outside and her house aflame. She stopped menstruating for eleven weeks.

Nor is it necessary for the stress to be so unpleasant: it can just as easily happen following happy circumstances.

YVONNE, a 25-year-old graphic artist, had a wonderful romance on a Greek island and stopped menstruating for nine weeks after she returned.

In both these cases it was the result of messages from the brain affecting the menstrual clock situated in the hypothalamus.

Factors which alter the other controlling centres in the hypothalamus (see Fig. 21) will also upset the menstrual clock. Common among these are rapid weight changes, especially anorexia nervosa or even rigid dieting which does not quite reach the proportions of anorexia nervosa. Each woman has her own critical weight level; if her weight falls below this then menstruation will stop and will not return until her weight returns to the critical level. Therefore those with a tendency to weight loss and missed menstruation are advised to weigh themselves each time menstruation occurs so as to learn their own personal weight limits. Depressive illnesses are also likely to delay menstruation, and again it is unlikely to return naturally until the depression is a thing of the past. Other chronic systemic illnesses, such as tuberculosis and acute rheumatic fever, can halt menstruation temporarily.

Lack of menstruation after stopping the pill may be an example where the ovary has been prevented from ovulating for so long that the menstrual clock has also been halted, and even when the pill is no longer being taken the menstrual clock does not restart automatically. More often there has been a weight loss during the time when the pill was being taken and on stopping the pill the weight loss amenorrhoea is revealed. Often when menstruation does restart after a long interval, the cycles are found to be anovular. This indicates that ovulation has not restarted although menstruation has, and a pregnancy is therefore impossible. Fortunately, nowadays, this can be corrected by appropriate hormone treatment.

Too Much

Menorrhagia is when menstruation goes on for too long, comes too often or is too heavy – in short when there is too much of it. Again stress can be the cause, although never in those women who on other occasions miss their menstruation at times of stress.

ZENA, *the 45-year-old wife of a TV producer, bled for nine weeks continuously, starting on the day her dream house, on which she had already put a deposit, was sold to a higher bidder without her knowledge.*

There is an interesting example in Mark's Gospel:

'And there was a woman who had a flow of blood for twelve years, and who had suffered much under many physicians, and had spent all that she had, and was no better, but rather grew worse. She had heard the reports about Jesus, and came up behind him in the crowd and touched his garment. For she said, "If I touch even his garments, I shall be made well." And immediately the haemorrhage ceased, and she felt in her body that she was healed of her disease.' (5, 25–59, RSV)

This incident can be seen in the light of our present medical knowledge. This woman had faith, and the tremendous emotional stress of being able actually to go up and touch the clothes that Jesus was wearing was sufficient stimulus to her menstrual clock to correct her prolonged menstruation.

Hormone therapy, as when taking the pill, and more especially the progestogen-only pill, may cause prolonged breakthrough bleeding, which can be a great nuisance and is a sign that treatment needs adjusting.

Occasionally there may be bleeding at ovulation; this is usually lighter and only lasts an hour or two or one or two days, but if there is no regular record of the bleeding it may not be easily recognized. A menstrual chart will clearly show the difference between the regular mid-cycle bleeding, which is harmless, and the totally irregular bleeding which needs gynaecological investigation.

Conditions which increase the surface area of the lining of the womb will result in heavy or prolonged bleeding. Examples are polyps, or fibroids which are situated near the cavity of the womb. However, as there is always the chance that the extra bleeding may be the result of a cancerous condition you are always justified in asking for a full examination.

Occasionally an intra-uterine device, whether a coil, loop or copper seven, may cause excessive bleeding or prolonged scanty bleeding for several days before and after menstruation. Although hormone treatment may be tried to stop the excessive bleeding, it is often best to remove the device and reinsert another in a more comfortable position in the womb. Sometimes a device has been in for years without any trouble, and then gradually menstruation gets more prolonged. This is usually a sign that the device is starting to dislodge and may indeed be pushed out of the womb into the vagina.

Sometimes the bleeding which is thought to be menstrual is due to the bleeding of an ulcer, or erosion, at the cervix or the opening to the womb. This can easily be spotted by a doctor on examination and he may well cauterize it.

18

The Vacant Plot

Can anyone blame the woman who for years has endured wretched miseries each month if she dreams of the day when those troublesome organs are removed by one clean swoop of the surgeon's knife? Already it is such a commonplace procedure in America that it is known as the Birthday Operation to be celebrated during the 40th year. Today the operative risks associated with the removal of the womb are minimal, but is it really an answer to a woman's prayers?

It is no good asking the gynaecologist, for he sees the woman a few months later, examines the scar to ensure it's well healed, assures her that she'll never again menstruate, possibly prescribes some oestrogen tablets, and says goodbye. It is better to ask the family doctor, who cares for this woman not just for one year but for the next twenty.

There are many very good reasons for the removal of the womb, and possibly the ovaries as well. At the top of that list would come any possibility of malignancy and no doctor will disagree here. Sometimes it is performed because of fibroids, either when they are so large that they are interfering with some other organ, or so numerous that they cause heavy menstruation resulting in anaemia; or because of endometriosis, and again these cases are certainly justified. On the other end of the scale there are those women who demand a hysterectomy so as to be 100% contraceptively safe, probably feeling that they cannot run the very small risk that exists with the pill or a device, or possibly having already tried these methods without success. A 42-year-old owner of a boutique confessed that she changed her gynaecologist seven times before she found one prepared to remove her womb merely for contraception. She stated that she was not convinced that sterilization would be reliable enough.

Far too many women have the operation in order to overcome their premenstrual syndrome. They would be better advised to have this condition treated with progesterone therapy. No one will disagree that on many occasions the symptoms are so severe that drastic treatment is warranted, but unfortunately a hysterectomy is not the answer. One well-known gynaecologist in London diagnoses premenstrual syndrome, explains to the woman that it is due to progesterone deficiency, does a hysterectomy and then refers her to the Premenstrual Syndrome Clinic for progesterone treatment.

Many of the problems for which the operation is recommended could alternatively be treated much more successfully with hormone therapy.

The immediate post-operative weeks are usually good and uneventful, but whether the womb only, or the womb plus the ovaries are removed, there is still an irreparable break in the hormonal pathway (Fig. 22) and the menstrual clock, which is not touched at operation, receives a severe jolt. Within six to eight days there is an increase in follicle stimulating hormone (FSH) from the pituitary and within eight to ten days an increase in luteinizing hormone (LH). The menstrual clock is reacting to the lack of information from the womb, and within a further three weeks there is a threefold increase in follicle stimulating hormone and a twofold increase in luteinizing hormone. This occurs whether or not the ovaries have been removed, although the increase is not so great if an oestrogen implant is given at the time of the operation.

The changes which occur with the surgical removal of the womb or ovaries are known as an 'artificial' menopause, and should not be confused with the natural menopause. In a natural menopause, the changes are very gradual over several years, with a slow closing down of the menstrual clock and shrinking of the ovaries and womb, but in an artificial menopause the changes are sudden and only affect the womb and/or the ovaries, leaving the menstrual clock intact.

All goes well after the operation for some 6–12 months, but then the difference between the two hormonal groups of women discussed on pages 162–3 begins to show itself. Those who previously suffered from the premenstrual syndrome will find that the usual cyclical symptoms return. Often it is the husband who is the first to notice it and he will try to remind the wife of what is happening. Or she may recognize the tell-tale headache, which previously ushered in a period and now assumes the proportions of a prostrating migraine.

> ANGELA, 48-year-old wife of a Squadron Leader, had a successful hysterectomy for fibroids which were causing heavy bleeding. She made an excellent recovery and assumed full household duties until nine months later, when she suddenly had four days of extreme tiredness. She stayed in bed attributing it to 'flu or some nasty virus. The following month it recurred, but this time she stayed in bed for six days. Gradually the duration of the tiredness lengthened until it represented two weeks in each month. It would start gradually with mere tiredness and she would manage to keep up for a few days, but then bed became essential. The end of the attacks was quite definite, and afterwards she had no other symptoms and resumed her normal social life.
>
> Her husband had kept a meticulous diary, from which a chart was constructed. When first seen she had already had nine months of this distressing condition, which fortunately responded completely to progesterone treatment.

Invariably premenstrual syndrome is more marked after a hysterectomy than before, and there may also be extra symptoms.

One woman, a part-time worker, was first seen at the police station after she had been charged with shoplifting. Two years previously a hysterectomy had been carried out. Prior to the operation she had suffered from premenstrual tension and headaches. After the operation her premenstrual syndrome had increased in severity and for a few days each month she would also experience breast fullness and a distressing feeling of unreality and confusion. She related these episodes to the time of her expected premenstruum and carefully charted the days on a calendar. She even went so far as to arrange her working days so as to avoid these inevitable confused days. In Court she described these days of confusion, explaining that sometimes she would come home having bought items she did not need, such as dog food when she had no dogs, curry and other foods which she never ate, and undies which were the wrong size. She was in a daze and could not recall what had happened. The day of her offence had been such a day. Even when she was taken to the police station by a plainclothes policeman after having been charged, she thought the officer was a rapist driving down an unknown road. The case was dismissed. She has since been under progesterone treatment, and is now free from cyclical confusion and premenstrual syndrome.

While carrying out a nationwide survey into the hormonal factors in migraine in women in 1975, it was noted that it was those women with a history of premenstrual syndrome who stated that the severity of their migraine had been increased by the hysterectomy. Their three-month charts giving the precise timing of migraine attacks confirmed that attacks were still occurring cyclically.

One cannot emphasize too strongly the need for women with cyclical symptoms to keep a careful record of their problem days, even if they have had their womb or ovaries removed. Sometimes when women feel very depressed and unable to record their days of depression, because the onset is so gradual, it is just as useful for them to record days on which they have breast symptoms, as these are usually very definite and commonplace. Alternatively, they can just record the days when they are feeling well with a tick.

> BRENDA, 47 years old, began her consultation with a detailed account of how her husband had been moved from Southern England to Lincolnshire, how she had made a suicide attempt within days of arriving there and had been hospitalized for several months. Within a week or two of her discharge she moved back to her previous village in the South of England, but made another suicide attempt the following week and was again admitted to hospital. It was only after compiling a long and confused history, assisted by her husband, that mention was made of a hysterectomy and the fact that she was now experiencing cyclical attacks of depression and moodiness. Once the cyclical nature of her symptoms was appreciated and confirmed by a two-month record it was possible to give her progesterone treatment and restore her to normality.

Two recent surveys have emphasized the high incidence of depression occurring in women one to three years after a hysterectomy, with or without the removal of the ovaries. The depression appears to be greatest in those under 40 years at the time of the operation; those with a previous history of depression, especially postnatal depression; those in whom no gynaecological abnormality could be found by the pathologist who examined the womb after operation (in one of the surveys 45% of the wombs were reported to be normal); and in those women who had a history of marital disruption.

Dr Donald Richards, a general practitioner in Oxford, realized that those patients who had previously had a hysterectomy were the patients whose medical notes were bulging out of their files so that at a glance one realized they had already done the rounds of most hospital departments. His survey, confirmed by others, emphasized the high incidence of depression in those with a history of a hysterectomy.

My paper on 'The Aftermath of Hysterectomy', read at the

Royal Society of Medicine in London in 1957, revealed that 44% of women had either been divorced, separated or had sought the assistance of a marriage-guidance counsellor since the operation. When the woman is ill each month with menstrual problems the husband is more sympathetic than he is when, after the operation, she flies into rages for no apparently accountable reason. One husband said, 'She used to have a reason for it, but now she's quite unpredictable,' and another, 'I hoped the operation would make her more even tempered.'

Another disturbing finding in the survey was that more than half of the women gained more than 28 lb. in the year following their hysterectomy. How often is a woman warned before the operation that the odds are two to one that such a marked weight-gain might occur? The reason for the depression and weight-gain after hysterectomy may be appreciated by recognizing the proximity of the menstrual clock to the mood controlling centre and the weight controlling centre in the hypothalamus (Fig. 21).

There would seem to be two types of post-hysterectomy depression, a cyclical depression and a continuous depression. The continuous depression is likely to be suffered by those who in their youth experienced spasmodic dysmenorrhoea and have a tendency to be oestrogen deficient. These women respond perfectly to oestrogen therapy, which needs to be continued not only until their depressive illness is past but well after the time of the natural menopause. The oestrogen is given continuously as there is no risk of it causing a build-up of the lining of the womb. If the depression is cyclical it will respond to progesterone. This should also be given continuously, even if ovulation is occurring, for there is no longer the possibility of causing irregularity of menstruation.

If it is only a hysterectomy that has been performed ovulation will continue, but with the interruption of the hormonal pathway there may be a gradual deterioration of ovarian function and a premature menopause. In such cases, as well as in those who have had their ovaries removed, there may be a decrease in bone mass with a risk of developing brittle bone disease, or osteoporosis. These women need hormone replacement therapy as well as an appreciation of the importance of calcium in their diet and the beneficial effect of moderate daily exercise.

A few women are found to have a high prolactin level, suggesting that the operation has caused a disturbance in the hypothalamic-pituitary mechanism. These women respond well to bromocriptine, a drug which lowers the prolactin level.

In theory the removal of the womb should have no effect on subsequent sexual activity – in fact it should be enhanced once the fear of a possible pregnancy is permanently removed. The vagina and clitoris are untouched at operation. In practice there are those who previously had a satisfactory sex life, and now suddenly find they have lost all urge and satisfaction. If this occurs it is well worth seeking professional help. Often testosterone is the magical restorative.

Perhaps it is relevant to mention that when apes have had their wombs removed their partners also reject them, but if the ape has only been given a mock operation, without the womb being removed, the couple enjoy a natural sexual relationship. Whether a similar effect occurs in humans is not yet known; one can only speculate.

Menopausal Years

It is only children who long to grow old. Adults hate the thought of it. This is never more true than when the menopause approaches, for this may be seen as a door leading to senility, when it is really the gateway to an era of serenity, for the postmenopausal years are characterized by confidence, calmness, sophistication, stable mood and endless energy.

Women are unique in the animal kingdom as the only females who outlive their reproductive function and can enjoy up to half their life span without it. The end of menstruation occurs according to an individual pre-arranged plan. The menstrual clock runs at its own individual rate; in some it runs on a little longer and in others it stops earlier.

Actually, the word 'menopause' means the pausing of menstruation, and more precisely, the last menstruation. It is the reverse of the menarche, but it cannot be timed as accurately because it is only seen in retrospect. Only when there have been no further menstruations for a year, can it be dated exactly. The term 'climacteric' was used to cover the years before and after the last menstruation, a time when the changes in the reproductive system were occurring, but nowadays it is usual to use the term 'menopause' more loosely to cover these years of hormonal change.

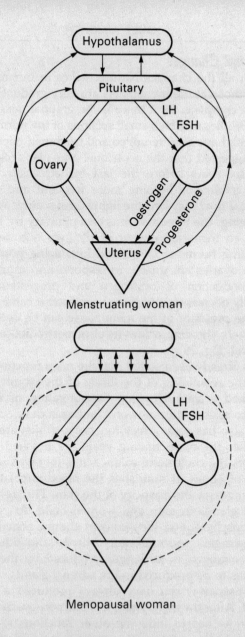

Fig. 29 Hormonal pathways in menstruating and menopausal women

Hormonal Changes

As with all the changes Nature makes in our reproductive system those at the menopause are very gradual, taking 5–7 years to complete. First there is the gradual missing of ovulation. Studies in which small sections of the normal lining of the womb have been removed and examined microscopically have suggested that the occasional anovular cycle can occur up to six years before the last menstruation. Gradually, missed ovulations become more frequent and with it the menstrual flow may become lighter and scanty. As the ovary is declining, the hypothalamus and pituitary try to stimulate it with an increased output of the two hormones, follicle stimulating hormone (FSH) and luteinizing hormone (LH). But the ovaries are unable to respond and cannot increase their production of oestrogen and progesterone, which gradually decreases until some years later it comes to an end. Thus the presence of the menopause can be determined by blood tests showing a low level of oestradiol and a raised FSH level (Fig. 29).

It has already been stated that the main function of oestrogen is the rebuilding of the lining of the womb after it has been shed at menstruation, the alteration of the cervical mucus to assist fertilization and for breast development. Oestrogen also has some other functions, which are of importance after the menstruating years are finished. Oestrogen promotes the cholesterol balance, it is involved in the building up of bones, it nourishes the blood circulatory system and it increases the elasticity of the skin. Throughout life the adrenal glands in men and women build up progesterone from cholesterol and then convert the progesterone further into oestrogen, testosterone, cortisone and other steroids. When oestrogen is no longer produced by the ovaries, it continues to be produced in the adrenal glands, and in peripheral tissues which have always produced a very small amount. After the menopause it is this non-ovarian oestrogen which now has to fulfil the other functions to the blood, bones and skin. All too often there is insufficient oestrogen for these other tasks, either temporarily during the change-

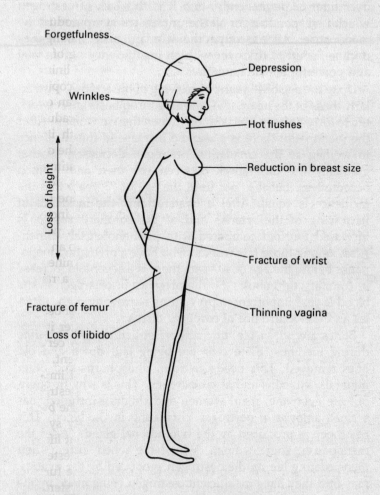

Forgetfulness

Depression

Wrinkles

Hot flushes

Reduction in breast size

Loss of height

Fracture of wrist

Fracture of femur

Thinning vagina

Loss of libido

Fig. 30 Oestrogen deficiency at the menopause

over time or permanently, and it is this lack of oestrogen which is responsible for all the unpleasant symptoms of the menopause. All too often the woman, once her ovaries decline, is left to tick over with an insufficiency of this vital and powerful female hormone.

Up to the age of 40 years, narrowing of the arteries, particularly those of the heart, and coronary thrombosis are between ten to forty times more common in men than in women. After the menopause there is a marked increase in this incidence in women as the circulating oestrogen decreases, so that gradually the differences between the men and women become less, but it is not until the age of 75 years that the incidence is equal. After a hysterectomy the incidence of narrowing of the arteries and of the coronary vessels is increased fourfold compared with premenopausal women. Also, among those few women who have a premature menopause before the age of 40 years there is a sevenfold increase in coronary thrombosis. So the presence of oestrogen in the blood is very important in preventing narrowing of the arteries and the occurrence of coronary disease.

Bones are not stable, unchanging structures. All the time during life, new bone cells are being laid down and old ones removed. This needs calcium, phosphorus and other minerals, vitamins and also oestrogen. This is why throughout life everyone, men, women and children included, has a small amount of oestrogen circulating in the blood. This oestrogen is produced by the two adrenal glands. After the menopause, some women, who have relied during their menstruating life on the oestrogen produced by the ovaries, may find they have insufficient oestrogen being made by the adrenals and this leads to thinning of the bones. This thinning of the bones shows up on X-rays, and ten years after the menopause it is present in 40% of all women. Although this can be halted with oestrogen administration, it takes another ten years before the X-rays show any improvement. Recent exciting work is showing that, while oestrogen halts bone deterioration after the menopause, progesterone is possibly more beneficial in building up bone mineral loss in post-hysterectomy women and at the menopause.

Progesterone is not required any more to prepare the lining of the womb or the cervical mucus for possible pregnancy after menstruation ceases, but progesterone also has another function. All through life, in both sexes, progesterone is also built up in the adrenal glands from cholesterol, and then immediately converted into oestrogen, testosterone, cortisone and other adrenal hormones, or corticosteroids, which have many and various jobs to do throughout the body. However, as ovarian progesterone was only present in the bloodstream for half of each cycle, the adrenals generally managed to make sufficient for their own needs during the menstruating years, and so they are usually capable of carrying on this task after the menopause. This is why after the menopause progesterone deficiency is no longer a problem, although if progesterone is given it can be converted into oestrogen.

Two Hormonal Groups

Earlier the two hormonal groups, the oestrogen-deficient and progesterone-deficient, were discussed, but apart from spasmodic dysmenorrhoea most of the previous chapters have dealt with the progesterone-deficient group and the havoc that can be caused by premenstrual syndrome in the home, at work and at leisure. At the menopause we again return to the oestrogen-deficient group, for these are the women whose menopausal sufferings begin earliest and are the most severe. This can be seen in Fig. 31, which shows that those women who had spasmodic dysmenorrhoea in their teens and then sufficient oestrogen for normal menstruation, nevertheless suffer most from menopausal symptoms; indeed, the chances are that they will be experiencing menopausal symptoms while their menstruation is still regularly occurring each month. Their need for oestrogen therapy at the menopause is essential and they are the ones who will probably need it for many years to come. Those who were

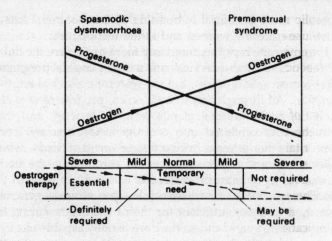

Fig. 31 Need for oestrogen therapy at the menopause

in the normal category may require oestrogen therapy during the changeover period, but they will then probably manage to make sufficient for their own requirements. The sufferers of mild premenstrual syndrome may require oestrogen temporarily when their menstruations first stop, but should gradually manage without. On the other hand the severe premenstrual syndrome sufferers are those who will probably have no need for oestrogen either during the menopausal years or later, since these women have always managed to have a high oestrogen level by supplementing the ovarian oestrogen with that which is produced in the adrenals.

In short it is a case of roundabouts and swings. Those who had greatest difficulties with monthly problems can look forward to a problem-free era, whilst those who had little trouble during the twenties and thirties are the ones with most problems at the menopause.

It will be noted that the term 'Hormone Replacement Treatment', or HRT, has been avoided because this only leads to confusion, for both oestrogen and progesterone are hormones and both are used in replacement therapy. But in the public mind and in the media HRT has become limited to the use of oestrogen therapy in the menopause. Hormone replacement therapy has been used for years in giving insulin to diabetics and thyroxine to those with an underactive thyroid.

Age of Menopause

In the United States the age of the menopause is 52 years; in Britain it is 48 years, with a range between 45 and 55 years. Those whose menstruation ceased before 45 years are said to have a 'premature menopause'.

The exact time of the menopause is very individual. However, a study of the following four factors can give some indication as to whether it is likely to be early or late:

- 1 The age of menarche. The effect of this is that those who start menstruation early tend to finish late, giving a 'rainbow' effect as shown in Fig. 32.
- 2 The hormonal group. Those in the oestrogen-deficient group have a tendency to finish menstru-

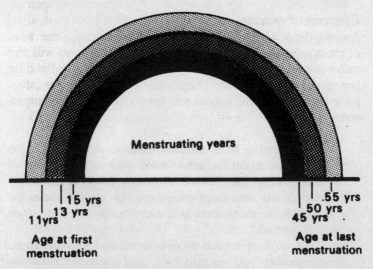

Fig. 32 Age of menarche and menopause

ation before the average, while sufferers from the premenstrual syndrome tend to finish after 50 years of age.

- 3 Genetic factor. Some families give a story of the mother, sister and aunts all finishing menstruation early, in which case such a patient may also expect to finish early. It is worth finding out at what age the patient's mother had her last normal menstruation. If your mother had an easy change of life the chances are that you are likely to have an easy time too. If she suffered, make sure you receive the benefit of modern medicine.

- 4 Smoking. A survey at the BUPA Medical Centre in London showed that at 48–49 years 36% of smokers were post-menopausal compared with 23% non-smokers; four years later the figures were 89% smokers and 71% non-smokers. So smoking habits should also be considered when estimating the probable age at which the menopause may occur.

Patterns of ending

Among those women who are regularly recording the dates of their menstruation, it can be seen that the menstruating years end in a wide variety of ways. Three patterns of ending are recognized, but even then some women may find that their own individual experience covers more than one pattern:

- 1 There may be a gradual ending, so that whereas menstruation initially lasted four or five days, it gradually lasts one or two days, then only one day or even one hour monthly, but nevertheless the cycle is maintained and menstruation comes when expected.

- 2 There may be the occasional missed menstruation, possibly just an odd one, and then menstruation resumes again for a month or two before another is missed; gradually there are more missed menstruations than actual menstruations, but each menstruation lasts the expected number of days, say four to six days.

- 3 There is the sudden ending of menstruation, which had previously been regular, the final menstruation lasting the normal or nearly normal number of days. This abrupt ending is more likely if it has coincided with a stressful event, such as a daughter's wedding, moving house, or becoming a grandparent. This abrupt ending may even be the start of a depressive illness.

The individual woman's attitude to a missed or delayed menstruation depends upon her recent sexual activity and desire for pregnancy. If there has been no sexual activity she may not notice the infrequency or absence of menstrual bleeding for a month or two; but if the possibility of pregnancy exists her attitude changes to one of concern with increasing happiness or unhappiness as each additional day of missed menstruation passes and confirms the diagnosis. The possibility of pregnancy is usually uppermost in the minds of those whose regular menstruation suddenly ceases. While pregnancy is the commonest cause in the earlier years, one must always first consider the possibility of the menopause after 45 years of age. Comments by patients in this predicament include:

'I don't want to get my name in the Guinness Book of Records as the oldest mum in the world.'

'I would hate to be drawing my old age pension when my child is still at school.'

and from a grandmother:

'My child would then be younger than her niece.'

Usually it is quite easy for a doctor to tell if a patient is pregnant or undergoing the menopause. If she is pregnant her breasts will be full, she may have symptoms of early-morning sickness and of passing urine during the night, and on examination her vagina is red and moist and the neck of the womb soft. On the other hand if she is entering the menopause her breasts will begin to decrease in size and firmness, she may have menopausal symptoms, especially flushes, and on examination her vagina will be pale and dry, and the neck of the womb firm and smaller.

Menopausal Flushes

The most characteristic symptom of the menopause is the 'hot flush', or 'flash' as it is called in America. It is a sensation of burning heat, arising from the waist and passing up to the top of the head. It only lasts a few minutes, five minutes at the most, and may be either visible, when the skin is flushed and beads of sweat appear, or it may be invisible. Very few women indeed pass through the menopausal years entirely without experiencing a single flush; they may range in frequency from only one or two a week to between fifty and a hundred a day. Many women are embarrassed by them, but others, working with women of their own age, giggle about them believing that 'a flush shared is a flush halved'. Our grandparents used to say that they were worth 'a guinea a flush'. They may be accompanied by palpitations, fluttering in the chest, or a feeling of choking, apprehension or anxiety. Flushes are worse immediately after a hot drink or spicy foods. If the flushes last longer than half an hour then there is likely to be some other cause for them.

The flushes can occur at night, when the woman usually awakes abruptly in a bath of sweat; these are known as 'night sweats'. When the wife awakes suddenly, flinging off the bedclothes, the husband is very likely to be annoyed rather than sympathetic.

A story is told about a group of women undergraduates at Girton College, Cambridge, in the twenties, who were discussing the menopausal problems and hot flushes that were being experienced by their parents and tutors. They agreed that as they were all so emancipated and fully understood the facts of life they would never have to suffer the ordeal of flushes. They formed a Menopause Club, promising to keep in touch with each other and give full accounts of how they fared through that great age. When the time came, each of them experienced the flushes and other menopausal symptoms to a greater or lesser extent, in spite of their full knowledge of the events of life.

It would seem that the flushes are due to a sudden stimulus in the temperature-controlling centre in the hypothalamus and are associated with a rise in the follicle stimulating hormone and luteinizing hormone from the pituitary gland as well as a deficiency of oestrogen.

Menopausal Symptoms

The symptoms are usually divided into two groups: the specific symptoms, which are due to deficient oestrogen and can be relieved by giving oestrogen, and the vague psychological symptoms, some of which may be relieved by oestrogen and some not, depending on the individual patient. Non-specific symptoms include tiredness, insomnia, irritability, depression, headaches, palpitations, anxiety, giddiness, forgetfulness and absentmindedness (Fig. 30, page 177). The psychological symptoms may represent a secondary result of the primary oestrogen deficiency symptoms, the so-called 'domino effect'. Thus the flushes, sweats, painful intercourse and nocturnal frequency of micturition may cause insomnia and subsequent tiredness and irritability.

Hot flushes and sweats are usually the first signs of oestrogen deficiency. Lack of oestrogen may cause the vagina to become dry, pale, thin and less resilient. There is a change in the acidity of the vagina which leads to a change in the bacterial flora of the vagina and a tendency to atrophic vaginitis and to infection, which in turn may cause itching, pain or frequency in passing urine especially at night, often misdiagnosed as cystitis. There is pain on initial penetration at intercourse and ultimately loss of sex urge.

The skin becomes pale and thinner, it loses its elasticity so that wrinkles develop, especially on the face around the eyes and mouth, and in the neck. The soaring sales of cosmetics, beauty treatments and the demand for cosmetic surgery are evidence of the obvious distress caused by these middle-age symptoms.

The rheumaticky pains that develop in the bones, muscles and joints are due to the thinning of the bones. There is often marked stiffness on rising in the mornings, and the pains tend to move about from one site to another over the course of weeks. Sometimes the joints of the fingers may become very painful, with marked swelling and then as the pain and swelling ease, the joint may be left deformed and 'out of true'. These vague generalized joint pains may represent the early sign of thinning of the bone mass, or osteoporosis, and suggest that in the postmenopausal years fractures of the wrist, neck of the femur and crushed fractures of the spine are likely to occur. The dowager's hump at the top of the spine is also a sign of thinning of the bones, but this does not develop until the seventies.

The thinning of the bones also causes a decrease in body height. Leonardo da Vinci in his 'Universal Man' demonstrated that the height equals the armspan, and so it is for men and premenopausal women. However, as a woman's vertebrae and discs become thinner after the menopause there is a decrease in height with no corresponding decrease in armspan. If there is more than 3 cm. loss of height compared with armspan it is an indication that the woman should be on long-term oestrogen therapy (Fig. 33).

The greatest bone loss occurs when menstruation is altering, becoming irregular and scanty, and during the two years after the last ever menstruation, and then the bone loss gradually decreases over the next twenty years. During these menopausal years the bones become thinner and osteoporosis starts. Gradually the changes lead to the 'little old lady' syndrome, 'little' because the height is lost, fat is reduced and possibly there is a dowager's hump, and 'old' because they are postmenopausal, and 'lady' because the development of osteoporosis is about five times more common in women than in men. This all results from the loss of oestrogen and progesterone, but there is much that can be done to prevent it (see pages 204–8).

The worst symptoms are the non-specific ones which led to the following comments:

'I think I must be going insane.'

'I feel so harassed the whole world seems to be resting on my shoulders.'

'It's even tougher than pregnancy and labour.'

At menopause there are mood changes, which are continuous, not mood swings which last only a fortnight or so at a time and then are eased, temporarily at least. It may turn an easy-going type into a shrew, a highly strung individual into a crying lunatic, a happy-go-lucky woman into an overworked, restless, nagging bitch, and a spry housewife into an absent-minded professor, who puts the cat in the fridge and the milk on the doorstep. At this time the woman leaves the femininity rat-race and her personality factors become more important and possibly exaggerated.

Even the woman's shape alters as her breasts begin to sag and she develops a spare tyre and middle-age spread. There is also the tendency for the thin to become scraggy and the fat to become obese.

Diagnosis

The diagnosis is usually not difficult to make on clinical grounds. The hot flush is most characteristic, but it must not be forgotten that some anti-depressants can also cause flushes. The thin skin, the greying hair, the wrinkles, the dry vagina, and deformed fingers and toes are all tell-tale

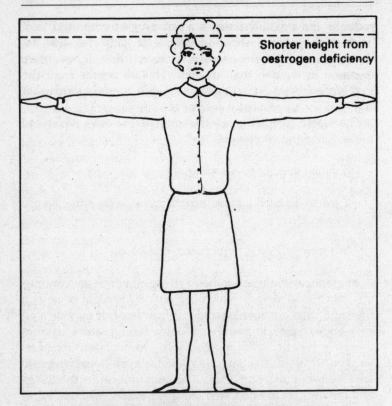

Normally the armspan equals the height, but if
oestrogen deficiency occurs at the menopause
the armspan exceeds the height

Fig. 33 Armspan equals height

signs. If further confirmation is needed a blood test will show
a rise in follicle stimulating hormone, and if the bones are
badly affected there will be a rise in blood calcium and phos-
phates. A simple test, which a doctor can do, is to examine
some of the vaginal cells under a microscope. The cells with
ample oestrogen have dark well-marked nuclei within them;
this is known as the Karyopicnotic Index (or KI) and is often
done routinely when a cervical smear is performed, but its

value is limited to the times when progesterone is absent, such as just after a period or after a long interval since the last period. If progesterone is present the cells lose their nuclei.

If the diagnosis is in doubt it is worth giving the woman a month's trial of oestrogen and if on her return she reports an improvement in the symptoms the prescription can be repeated. Admittedly there is frequently a beneficial placebo effect merely from giving the tablets, but if the benefit is still maintained two or three months later it strongly suggests that it is the hormone which is beneficial.

The effect of the menopause on sexual activity depends on one's experience during the menstruating years. If sex was important then it is likely to be even more enjoyable once the fear of pregnancy is permanently eradicated. If there was never much sexual excitement then many think of the menopause as a time when this activity may be slowed down or stopped. If oestrogen deficiency is present and making the vagina sore and coital penetration painful these symptoms can be easily relieved by giving oestrogen, either as a cream to be used locally or by tablets.

Those who talk and write, in error, of the 'male menopause' refer to it as a time when a man's sexual urge diminishes. This is nothing more than anti-chauvinism. It is regrettable because it gives the impression that this is what is happening to women at the menopause, which is quite wrong.

When Neurgarten was carrying out his study on the attitude to the menopause he asked the loaded question, 'What is the best thing about menopause?' to which 44% replied 'not having to bother about menstruation', 30% 'not being worried about getting pregnant' and 14% 'the better relationship with husband and greater enjoyment of sex life'.

The International Health Foundation in 1969 studied the subject and interviewed 2000 women between 45 and 55 years and 72% agreed that after the menopause it was good to be free from menstruation. The figures for the various countries ranged from 66% in Italy to 79% in the United Kingdom.

Empty Nest Syndrome

Unfortunately the menopausal years are often traumatic for women in other ways. It has been calculated that in the space of the five years around her fiftieth birthday, the average woman will lose her mother through death, her daughter through marriage and become a grandparent. There are also those whose children leave home for college or other employment, who move house or whose husband changes his job or receives his final promotion. This has led psychologists to refer to the 'empty nest syndrome', believing that all the miseries of menopausal symptoms are but a reaction to the woman's empty life. While some women may be upset by these events, and accepting that such events will cause emotional impulses to reach the menstrual clock, nevertheless in the vast majority of cases the menopausal symptoms have a hormonal basis and respond well to oestrogen therapy. Full details of treatment are to be found in Chapter 21.

20

Do It Yourself

There is a widespread hope that there may be some magic way of coping with monthly problems without having to disturb the busy doctor. Certainly in mild cases it is important to try to tackle the problems yourself, with the full knowledge that if you do not succeed, further help, and most effective help, is available from any doctor who understands hormone therapy.

First let us deal with the 'old wives' tales' and remind you that there's no truth in the idea that you mustn't have a bath, go swimming, or walk barefoot when you're menstruating or you will catch your death of cold. We now know that pneumonia and viral disease commonly starts during the premenstruum, which is probably how the idea began. It won't matter if you do wash your hair when you're menstruating, although some women with very fine hair may find that a set at this time of the month won't stay in for long, so if you're paying for an expensive set wait just a few days longer. Another tale is that taking a cold shower will reduce the menstrual flow. This is wrong for the menstrual flow is going to come away normally in its own good time.

The desire to 'do-it-yourself' came from a Community Nurse who wrote:

'I have always tended to be moody since my teens, but since my second pregnancy I have spells of hell, during

*which my doctor gives me tranquillizers. These help a bit,
but as a state registered nurse and health visitor you can
imagine my training screams out, "Treat the cause, not
the result." Please tell me what I can do to help myself.'*

And from another nurse who pleaded:

*'There must be something more – I don't just want to take
anti-depressants permanently when I feel so very well and
am perfectly OK for half the month.'*

Spasmodic Dysmenorrhoea

For those with spasmodic dysmenorrhoea, relaxation and
correct breathing is valuable, but unfortunately the benefit is
not so marked in those with premenstrual syndrome. It has
been mentioned earlier that the type of pain suffered by
those with severe spasmodic dysmenorrhoea is similar to
labour pains. Actually, the same nerves are involved in opening the door of the womb to let the baby out as are needed
at menstruation to open the door to let out the menstrual
flow. Nowadays it is universally recognized that in preparation for labour women benefit by relaxation exercises and
correct breathing. Gradually it is being appreciated that these
same relaxation exercises are of benefit to relieve the pain of
dysmenorrhoea. Some of our schools already teach their
older girls relaxation as part of physical education and sufferers from dysmenorrhoea have obtained much benefit from
this. Relaxation for Living is an organization in Britain which
exists purely to promote the teaching of relaxation, not only
for that one day when the woman is in labour, but to help
both men and women to relax during normal day-to-day
living. They also have a cassette tape to help those who
would prefer to learn relaxation in the cosiness of their own
home. The National Childbirth Trust runs classes throughout
Britain for those who are pregnant, and is usually most helpful in supplying the name of a local teacher who will help
either an individual or a group of women with dysmenorrhoea.

Drs Margaret Chesney and Donald Tasto compared the effects of relaxation on college students in California. The students were initially separated into those with spasmodic dysmenorrhoea and those with premenstrual syndrome; they were then divided into one of three treatment groups by drawing lots. One treatment group received relaxation treatment at five weekly sessions and were told to practise the exercises daily at home, another group attended a leaderless psychotherapy group where they compared each other's experiences of period pain for five weekly sessions, and the last group were left untreated on the waiting list. All students completed questionnaires dealing with the severity of their pain before treatment and for three cycles after treatment was completed. Those who had spasmodic dysmenorrhoea and took relaxation classes reported a dramatic improvement in their pain, which was sustained afterwards. So there does seem to be positive hope from simple treatment for those with spasmodic dysmenorrhoea. However, if one is still crippled with pain after thoroughly mastering the relaxation technique, there should be no hesitation in seeking help from the doctor.

Prostaglandin inhibitors are considered safe enough by the Committee on Safety of Medicines to be sold over the counter by chemists, so it is worthwhile having the advice of your chemist when choosing the most suitable one for you. If your cycle is regular it is best to start on half the dose for the four days before the pain is expected and then increase to full dose as soon as menstruation starts. An added bonus is that the total blood loss is usually reduced by an average of 25%.

It is advisable to keep a menstrual chart so that you know when next to expect menstruation, you can notice if the pain comes every month and if it has been improved by the simple measures suggested.

Premenstrual Syndrome

Sufferers from premenstrual syndrome will need different help. The first important thing is to keep a menstrual chart.

You can easily devise your own but it is better to use the
type shown in Fig. 3 (page 22); it is the records which are
important. If the chart shows the presence of symptoms
during the paramenstruum with freedom from symptoms
during another phase of the cycle, accept the diagnosis,
realize you're not alone but that some millions of other
women in Britain are suffering likewise. Many letters
received after a television programme entitled *Pull Yourself
Together, Woman* expressed this sense of relief at knowing
they were not alone in their suffering:

> *'I went to sleep happy that night knowing that I was not
> alone in my suffering.'*

> *'Just to know I wasn't mad. I never dared talk about it, I
> thought I was the only one.'*

> *'All my problems were so peculiar I didn't expect anyone
> else to understand.'*

What's more you might even try charting a friend's problems, such as colds, breakages, or temper tantrums. Some
people have complaints month after month and never link it
up or make the connection with menstruation. They merely
announce, 'I've got another cold.'

Having accepted the diagnosis yourself, talk about it. First
your husband should know and understand so that he is
able to help you. Wait until you feel well and then tell him
how unhappy you feel about your periodic loss of control,
and, if it is relevant, about your fears that you might one
day harm your baby or attempt an overdose. As mentioned
earlier, sometimes when you feel most bloody-minded you
nevertheless have an increased sex urge during the premenstruum; discuss it with him, explain your difficulties, tell him
that you know you're being horrid but you can't help it and
you still love him and want him to love you. Having realized
that there's nothing of which to be ashamed, talk to the other
people with whom you come into contact so that they may

be able to understand you better. Discuss it with your friends so that they can appreciate your difficulties and stand by you. Explain to your workmates and to your in-laws, and don't forget it is just as important that men understand as well. Above all see that your adolescent children understand and accept all that it entails. If you are at school, you should discuss it with your teacher, or if you are too shy you may like your mother to speak to her instead.

During a Sunday family dinner my adolescent daughter broke a plate when she was clearing away the first course. 'Don't worry, it's the wrong day of the month,' commented my son. Not many minutes later my other daughter knocked over a glass and broke it. Trying to clear up the mess I knocked over a bowl of vegetables on to the floor. 'I think we men will have to take care of the washing-up today,' remarked my other son calmly. It seemed a far better way of dealing with a biological disturbance, rather than scolding the two girls for their apparent clumsiness and breakages.

Mark in your diary when you may expect your next period. Don't just count 28 days because others have a cycle of 28 days, but count the days of your last cycle and mark in the correct number of days for you personally. Consult your diary before arranging your next dinner party; avoid those awkward days if you have an interview, an examination or driving test. Arrange to have your permanent wave or tint during the postmenstrual week, it'll take better then. If you're a journalist don't accept a deadline for any article which will clash with the worst time of the month. School-teachers in the upper school can just as easily set homework two weeks ahead so that the girls can do it when in their postmenstrual peak. If you have to take examinations when you're feeling ill, make sure you tell the invigilator and he will write a note on your paper telling the examiner.

If you're at work tell your employer or your personnel manager. It helps if they understand. If flexitime is worked at your office you'll be able to keep some hours or days in hand to use when necessary. If there is shift work, try to get on the 2–10 shift, so that you've time to get up without

hurrying and dose yourself up before starting the day's work.
Sufferers from the premenstrual syndrome should, if possible, avoid night-shift working as nothing is more unsettling
for the menstrual clock than muddling night and day
(remember the 'sleep and waking' control centre is also in
the hypothalamus near the menstrual clock).

Eat Every Three Hours
On pages 154–6 the importance of the lower mechanism
for the control of blood sugar, is explained. This regulating
mechanism is raised premenstrually in sufferers of premenstrual syndrome and it is, therefore, vital to ensure that long
intervals without some starchy food are eliminated. The rule
is to have small portions frequently, every three hours.
Instead of having a slice or two of toast at breakfast, halve
it and save the other half to enjoy with the mid-morning
coffee. At lunch cut the sandwich (or whatever starchy food
you usually have) into two so that you have something to
eat with your afternoon tea. Save something from your evening meal to enjoy before going to bed. It's really quite easy
and there's no need to eat more than your usual quantity.

It is important to realize that whether or not you are going
to require progesterone therapy later, it is still essential to
continue with the three-hourly starch regime, so even if you
only think you might have premenstrual syndrome it is still
worthwhile starting on this eating regime while you're busy
keeping records.

By starchy food is meant anything made from flour,
potatoes, rye, oats and rice. This will therefore include bread,
biscuits, crispbread, crisps and cereal, but be fully aware
that it does *not* include fruit, bananas, cheese, chocolate and
yoghurt, which may be eaten with, but not instead of starchy
foods.

PMS Help, a non-profit-making charity which helps sufferers from premenstrual syndrome, promotes the three-
hourly starch rule and has produced a booklet on dietary
advice. In 1989 a survey among sufferers of premenstrual

syndrome asked whether they had a good, moderate or poor response to various treatments. Of the 250 replies 68% reported a good response to the three-hourly starch regime with only 1% giving a poor response. Of course such a treatment can only be advocated by a charitable organization as there is no financial gain to be had from the promoter. It is a regime which entails no financial outlay, but does demand self-discipline. One housewife rightly stated, 'I couldn't believe that the answer to all those ghastly PMS days lay in the kitchen.'

It is wise always to carry some emergency supplies of food in your handbag ready for that long wait in the queue or the slow journey home. If your children are over five tell them that Doctor says you must eat every three hours. It is amazing how cooperative children can be, always hoping that they too can enjoy a bite. Be sure that your husband understands too. It might help if you buy a watch which you can set to bleep every three hours, or at least an alarm clock if you're alone in the house all day. It is essential to keep to the frequent snacks right through the cycle; it is no good just limiting it to the premenstruum.

It is useful to complete an 'attack form', as shown in Fig. 14, whenever you have a sudden attack of irritability, panic, or headache. It is surprising how often such problems start when there has been a food interval exceeding three hours. Incidentally if you transgress and do inadvertently go too long without food, you may be surprised to find that it may take up to seven days to return to your normal level of fitness.

If you are good with your 'three-hour rule' it is not necessary to limit your liquids drastically. However, do not exceed two pints daily. It is also in order to eat the normal amount of salt, but don't overdo it. See that your diet contains proteins and plenty of fruit and vegetables.

If you're going to indulge in alcohol be warned that only half your usual amount will be required to make you merry. In sufferers from premenstrual syndrome, intoxication can easily occur during the paramenstruum. It's as well to consider the other golden rules with regard to alcohol. Don't mix grape and grain alcohol, or better still don't mix your drinks. Avoid drinking on an empty stomach and don't drink and drive.

If constipation is a problem, or if you're unfortunate enough to have irritable bowel syndrome, then it is wise to add a tablespoon of bran to your breakfast every day. That is not quite the same as bran flakes or bran cereals. It is the natural bran that is important, the stuff that looks and tastes like sawdust. It cannot be enjoyed alone, but can be mixed with your other cereals, added to fruit juice, yoghurt or stewed fruit. Make it a daily habit and after about two weeks you will appreciate the benefit with the regular, smooth opening of your bowels. In severe cases it may be necessary to have two tablespoons of bran daily, or have another helping at night with cereals, soup, jacket potato, stewed fruit or yoghurt.

There is no evidence that premenstrual syndrome is due to a poor diet or to a deficiency of any known vitamin or mineral. Problems due to nutritional deficiencies, which can occur in men and women of all ages, will be present throughout the month, although like all chronic diseases the symptoms may be worse during the paramenstruum. Vitamins and minerals have no place in the treatment of premenstrual syndrome in those enjoying a healthy diet. It is wise to avoid foods, particularly cereals, which have been 'enriched with vitamins'. This usually means vitamin B6 has been added, and, as explained on page 220, excess of vitamin B6 can result in neurological symptoms.

It's a good idea to give yourself extra rest during the second half of the cycle, and if necessary an afternoon nap too. Even if you don't go off to sleep, or into a state of semi-consciousness, it is resting in bed in the dark with the eyes shut that counts.

If a sufferer from premenstrual syndrome has taken all this advice and is still in trouble I would have no hesitation in suggesting a visit to the doctor, appreciating that he has help at hand especially for your problem. But remember to take your carefully prepared chart with you so that he, too, can confirm the diagnosis. It is wise to time the visit for the premenstruum.

Menopause

Throughout this chapter, simple do-it-yourself measures have been suggested for the treatment of menstrual problems. If these have failed, then it is suggested that medical advice should be sought. However, if menopausal symptoms are present it is advisable to seek medical advice sooner rather than later. Menopausal symptoms are due to oestrogen deficiency, and if this is allowed to continue it may lead to osteoporosis. At an early consultation your doctor will be able to assess your personal risk factors in developing osteoporosis, taking into account your family history, smoking, alcohol, exercise, previous amenorrhoea and your pill experience.

It is wise to avoid caffeine, hot drinks and spicy foods as these are liable to spark off hot flushes, and it is sensible to wear thin undies and nighties, preferably cotton ones to absorb the perspiration. If night sweats are a problem, then sheets and blankets are better than duvets, which keep the heat for so much longer. Before retiring it is worth having a starchy snack as sometimes the night sweats are caused by low sugar setting off an adrenalin spurt.

Your smoking habits and alcohol intake need consideration as these can hasten osteoporosis. It is also important to keep up some daily exercise. This does not just mean the normal walking to and fro while pottering about at home, but concentrated exercise for about twenty minutes, which leaves you breathless for at least five minutes. Choose what suits you best, either a good brisk walk daily, a daily swim, a game of tennis, skipping or using a bicycle machine in front of the TV each day while watching your favourite programme.

Think about your diet, and make sure you have sufficient calcium, which is in milk, cheese and fish, and that your daily intake of protein is adequate. It might be mentioned that there is more calcium in white than in wholemeal bread. Consider carefully if you need a weight-reducing diet, remembering that during these years of change the fat ones tend to get fatter and the thin ones become thinner. If you are already below the ideal weight for your age and height, don't make matters worse by reducing further, rather try to reach your personal ideal weight.

If the nights are very disturbed don't be ashamed of a short catnap after lunch. Your skin will also benefit from some cream to combat the natural dryness, and your greasy hair may need special shampoo.

21

How Can the Doctor Help?

'How I resent those eight years of suffering now I know how easy it is to cure.'

'If only others knew that operations and being admitted to hospital is not the answer to these beastly, savage changes of mood with the curse . . . the real treatment is so simple.'

The first step the doctor has to take when seeing a patient with menstrual problems is to ascertain the diagnosis, reassure himself that there is not some other accompanying disease, such as depressive illness, as well as premenstrual depression, and convince himself that there is no evidence of malignancy.

'My doctor treats all of us with a D & C and that's it.'

This comment may well be true, and merely shows how careful the doctor is being, in first eliminating the possibility of cancer in the body of the womb, which would not show up on a cervical smear or pap smear. On the other hand, many gynaecologists resort to the operation of dilatation and curettage at the drop of a hat, and such treatment can do nothing to cure any hormonal imbalance.

Having made sure of his diagnosis, the doctor now has to decide whether to use hormone therapy and, if so, which one. In this book we have been concerned essentially with the two menstrual hormones, oestrogen and progesterone. Earlier chapters have shown how a deficiency of either of them will result in a completely different presentation of symptoms. To give progesterone to a woman suffering from spasmodic dysmenorrhoea or menopausal symptoms will only make her worse, and the same happens when oestrogens are given for premenstrual syndrome. This is why a definite diagnosis is essential before treatment can begin. (See Chapter 3.)

Oestrogen Therapy

The first oestrogens to be used were non-steroid, which had completely different formulae from the natural ones found in the body. These included stilboestrol, dioenoestrol and hexoestradiol, which have been shown to have some cancer-producing potential and are never used for oral administration today, although dioenoestrol cream is sometimes recommended to be applied to the vagina. It is the natural oestrogens which are now prescribed. Their most important uses are in the treatment of spasmodic dysmenorrhoea, to help mature the womb in adolescence, at the menopause to substitute for the failing of the ovarian oestrogen, and in the contraceptive pill.

Spasmodic Dysmenorrhoea

For many years oestrogens were the standard treatment for spasmodic dysmenorrhoea. We now know that women suffering from this have high levels of prostaglandin F2 alpha. This knowledge has revolutionized treatment. Today the drugs of choice are prostaglandin inhibitors which decrease the amount of prostaglandin in the tissues. Some inhibitors are specific against prostaglandin F2 alpha while others are more effective in reducing the prostaglandin released when bone cells are damaged. Mefanamic acid, or Ponstan, is an effective prostaglandin inhibitor against F2 alpha and will both reduce the dysmenorrhoea and reduce the menstrual flow by about 25%. The tablets may be taken in half the dose (250 mg.) for the four days before the pain is expected and then increased to full dose, 500 mg. three times daily, as soon as menstruation starts and continued until the pain has ceased.

If oestrogen is being used it is given in courses from day 5 for 21 days, and menstruation usually occurs within two days of stopping the tablets. The first course will result in painless menstruation, because it has stopped ovulation for that month, but if one wants to remove spasmodic dysmenorrhoea permanently it is necessary to give many courses, perhaps for six to twelve months. In the sixties, when doing an investigation into period pains, it was surprising how many women wrote that they had received one course of oestrogens, which had only helped in that one month but made no difference thereafter. This is quite correct, but it is a shame it was not pointed out to the women, on starting treatment, that more than one course would be necessary to remove pain altogether.

The oestrogen can either be given alone or mixed with progestogens as in the oestrogen-progestogen pill. The advantage of giving the pill is that one is sure menstruation will occur after 21 days and of course the pills are prepared in carefully dated packs of 21 so that they are not so easily forgotten, or if forgotten the mistake is easily visible and two tablets can be taken at once when remembered. The advantage of giving oestrogen alone is that varying amounts can be given, thus allowing for individual differences. However, bleeding does not always occur at the end of the course. If oestrogen is used alone the woman must be fully aware that it is not a contraceptive.

DEIRDRE, 19 years, had been given oestrogen in Australia to relieve spasmodic dysmenorrhoea. She came to Britain on a six-month holiday complete with sufficient tablets to last her stay. After about four months she realized she had

missed her period and begun to develop morning sickness.
Her pregnancy test proved positive.

As she was taking a pill every day for three weeks and stopping for one week, like all her friends who were on an oral contraceptive, she assumed hers was also contraceptive.

Mothers are often upset by the thought that their daughters are being given the pill to ease period pains. They need to be reassured and told that this will not immediately lead their virgin daughters up the path of rampant promiscuity. The girls too need to be reassured that in spite of the terrible pains their fertility is good, and the very fact of pain shows that they are ovulating and so should not have much trouble in conceiving.

Occasionally women asking for treatment of spasmodic dysmenorrhoea are also anxious to begin a family. In these cases it is worth giving a higher dose of oestrogen from days 5 to 10 and days 18 to 28 of each cycle, avoiding oestrogen at the time of ovulation so that conception can occur.

When oestrogen is used for spasmodic dysmenorrhoea before 25 years of age, side effects are rare because there is insufficient oestrogen in the body. Contra-indications are hardly ever encountered in those with spasmodic dysmenorrhoea.

Oestrogens for Menopausal Symptoms

When oestrogens are given for menopausal symptoms the effect is dramatic. Within one week a marked lessening in the number of daily flushes may be expected, while if the flushes are still there in three weeks' time, it is a sign that a higher dose should be used. In Britain prescriptions for oestrogens have increased by 50% during the last several years, suggesting that their value is now being fully appreciated.

Women who are still menstruating can have oestrogen from day 5 until the time of their expected menstruation. While for many women this may mean a three-week course, those with longer cycles would be better to have a longer course of oestrogens, otherwise they may well have to go perhaps two weeks without treatment and risk the return of all their symptoms.

It is suspected that the build-up of the lining of the womb from oestrogen therapy in women who are not menstruating may be so marked that it might predispose to a risk of cancer. No one really knows whether this is so, but there is a ready answer to this problem which is worth considering. The lining can be shed by the addition of some progestogen tablets taken for a few days and then stopped. Bleeding is then likely to occur within a day or two of stopping. The progestogen can either be added to the oestrogen tablet and taken daily for three weeks and then stopped for a week during which bleeding will occur, or it need only be added for the last seven to ten days of the three-week course of oestrogen. However some women find the added progestogens cause premenstrual syndrome. These women benefit from the addition of natural progesterone suppositories, which can be used rectally or vaginally, rather than the artificial progestogens, which are alien to the human body. Progestogens are known to lower the blood level of progesterone, so it is not surprising that they cause symptoms of premenstrual syndrome. In France, but not in Britain, oral tablets of natural micronized progesterone are available, and as only a small amount of progesterone is required to provoke bleeding from an oestrogen-primed endometrium, oral progesterone is effective for this use.

On the other hand those women who have had the removal of their womb and are suffering from menopausal symptoms will also benefit from oestrogen therapy. They will not need to have the added progestogen as there is no risk whatsoever of them developing cancer of the womb.

Oestrogen can also be given by an implant, in which one or more small pellets of pure oestrogen are inserted, under the influence of a local anaesthetic, into the fat of the abdominal wall through a small incision in the skin. An implant means that the patient does not have the bother of trying to remember to take her daily tablets, but if any side effects develop it is not possible to remove the pellet. It is particularly useful in women with menopausal symptoms who have had a hysterectomy in the past. An oestrogen implant can also be performed for younger women during the course of their hysterectomy operation in order to prevent too great a shock to their menstrual hormonal pathway. If there is any loss of libido a pellet of testosterone may be implanted at the same time as the oestrogen pellet, with beneficial effect.

Oestrogen can also be absorbed through the skin and plasters are now available, which are applied to the lower abdomen and changed twice weekly. These have the advantage that the oestrogen does not pass through the liver but goes direct to the tissues requiring oestrogen, and so the side effects of oestrogen are diminished. It is still necessary to have regular vaginal bleeding if the woman has a womb, and this is given by the usual course of progestogen tablets.

The oestrogen replacement therapy should be continued until there are no symptoms when the oestrogen is stopped. If the woman is having a three-week course of oestrogen, and she notices slight flushes during the week without treatment, she is not yet ready to stop. If she is free from symptoms then she can leave it ten days before starting the next course, and if all goes well, fourteen days. If she can go three weeks without oestrogen it is a sign that her body has learnt how to make the necessary oestrogen for healthy bone metabolism and she can stop hormone replacement. Just how long it will be necessary to continue will vary with the individual woman, and there are an unlucky few who may need to continue for ten years or more.

It is still a vexed question among the medical profession whether or not there is any risk in prolonged oestrogen therapy. Certainly there does not appear to be a risk with short-term treatment of less than five years. Follow-up studies of women who have had oestrogen for fifteen or more years are difficult and confusing. In those days many women had the non-steroidal oestrogens which are known to carry a risk. We only hear of the cases where cancer develops, and we do not know whether this really represents all the women in the sample who have been having oestrogen for a long time. Even women who have never had oestrogen do develop cancer of the womb. Several long-term studies are in progress now, but it may be many years before the answer is available.

For their own safety and peace of mind women on oestrogen therapy should be seen at least every six months for a check on their blood pressure and weight, a breast and general examination, and a cervical smear.

The side effects of oestrogen are a feeling of nausea, bloatedness, headaches and depression, but these will only occur with women in whom there is no oestrogen deficiency, such as women with premenstrual syndrome. The side effects stop when oestrogen is stopped.

In Britain a ten-year breast cancer study involving 30,000 women is currently being carried out. It is designed to test whether the established anti-oestrogen drug, tamoxifen, which is used to treat breast cancer, might also protect women who are predisposed to the disease. It is estimated that if tamoxifen produces a 30% improvement in the incidence of breast cancer after it is taken for five years, the results will be detectable in ten years, while a 50% improvement will be detected in six years.

On the other hand, long-term oestrogen therapy has its benefits. The incidence in women of ischemic heart disease and strokes rises abruptly after menopause or after a hysterectomy or oophorectomy. It is likely that oestrogen therapy reduces this risk, although again this cannot be positively proven for a few years yet.

Some years ago at a meeting of a women's group where a talk was given on menopause one member of the audience was very vocal and anxious to tell the audience that her doctor had refused to give her oestrogen for her hot flushes. Later in the talk mention was made of the indications for avoiding giving oestrogens, which include a past history of coronary thrombosis, angina, pulmonary embolism, deep vein thrombosis, cancer of the breast, womb or ovary, diabetes, liver disease and high blood pressure. The same woman then rose and apologized as she was under treatment for high blood pressure. Today high blood pressure is no longer regarded as a contra-indication to oestrogen therapy, although the blood pressure would first need to be brought under control with our present effective hypotensive medication. It would be wiser to give oestrogen plasters rather than tablets, so bypassing the liver. In cases where oestrogen is definitely contra-indicated relief of symptoms and prevention of osteoporosis may be obtained from progesterone therapy, for progesterone is normally made in the adrenals where it is converted into oestrogen. Recent work has shown that progesterone is as effective as oestrogen, and possibly more effective, in preventing osteoporosis.

Some doctors feel that by eliminating the menstrual cycle they can thereby also eliminate premenstrual syndrome. Unfortunately, it is not as easy as that for, as we have noted, cyclical symptoms still occur after a hysterectomy and oophorectomy. Some advocate the insertion of an oestrogen implant to abolish menstruation, and then the addition of progestogens at the beginning of each month to ensure that there is regular shedding of the lining of the womb. The menstrual cycle of women who undergo such treatment is disturbed for up to one year and symptoms occur throughout the cycle. Their symptom-free postmenstruum is abolished.

Treatment for the Premenstrual Syndrome

A woman journalist conducted a small private survey to find out what doctors up and down the country were doing about menstrual problems. She noted the following as pretty standard answers:

> 'It (progesterone) doesn't work, and anyway everybody's on the pill.'

> 'It can only be given by injections.'

'There is no proof it works.'

'Placebo effects.'

*'Women are supposed to get some kind of masochistic plea-
sure from their pains.'*

There is nothing very surprising about these comments,
for they are typical of the attitudes which are delaying, for
many sufferers from premenstrual syndrome, the relief to
which they are entitled. The first one is typical of the confusion in many doctors' minds between progesterone and
progestogens. Progestogens do not work on premenstrual
syndrome but progesterone does. The confusion is reinforced
by the statement that follows, 'everybody's on the pill'. The
next comment is from those who certainly know the difference but are unaware of the progress that has been made
with suppositories and pessaries. The third remark is symptomatic of our scientific age which cannot accept the evidence
of its own eyes without the support of double blind trials.
'The proof of the pudding is in the eating,' or so it is said.
The ladies whose quotes appeared at the beginning of this
chapter needed no further proof of its value in treating premenstrual syndrome than their own happy experience. The
others need no comment and indeed they are all rather like
doctors' old wives' tales. But in fairness to the doctors it must
be remembered that not many who are practising today were
taught anything about these hormones or hormone receptors
when they were at medical school. However, today there are
increasing numbers of doctors who do know how and when
to use oestrogen and progesterone to remove the monthly
sufferings of women.

Progesterone

The first time the word 'progesterone' was used was by
Willard Allen, who with George Corner first isolated the
active constituent of the corpus luteum in the ovary. He

proposed the name in December 1934 and eight months later the principal scientists involved in the work on this new female sex hormone accepted the name. In 1943 Russell Marker emerged from the jungles of Central America and showed biochemists how to manufacture this pregnancy hormone, progesterone, from the roots of yams. However, once the biochemists had learnt the knack of manufacturing progesterone from yams its importance was overshadowed by the many other steroids that could be obtained from progesterone just by a subtle alteration of its chemical formulae. In their laboratories biochemists converted progesterone into the life-saving hormone, cortisone; it was also converted into progestogens, which are the basis of oral contraceptives used by countless women the world over (these synthetic progestogens are often mistaken for progesterone, but when taken by women they actually lower the progesterone level in the blood). Progesterone is also converted into oestrogens to satisfy the demand for hormone replacement therapy, and into testosterone for the restoration of male potency.

Progesterone Therapy

For many doctors progesterone is a forgotten hormone so far as treatment is concerned, and many doctors who use oestrogen, and know its possibilities and limitations, fight shy of using progesterone. One problem being that oral progesterone is not effective in the treatment of premenstrual syndrome, so it has to be given in other ways, such as pessaries, suppositories, injections or implants. In India, work on monkeys suggested that progesterone could be absorbed into the bloodstream when given by nasal administration, so aerosols and nasal sprays were tried, with little success. Later it was shown that progesterone cream applied to the nose of female rats was well absorbed. An American pharmaceutical company, 'Nastech', reported in 1985 that tests had been carried out on normal women in North Carolina, USA, and in Yorkshire, England, using progesterone nasal ointment with satisfactory results. There are hopes that this method of administration may revolutionize future progesterone therapy.

However, whenever progesterone therapy is necessary it is also essential that the patient follows the three-hourly starchy food regime discussed on pages 196–7. Like a diabetic on insulin (although insulin is the life-saver) who needs to stick to a strict diabetic diet, the premenstrual syndrome patient needs to stick to the three-hourly starch regime.

When women with premenstrual syndrome, who have been treated with progesterone, return to the doctor it is often difficult to recognize them as the same women who first came for advice and treatment. The woman, who has so often taken an overdose during the late premenstruum when life was on top of her, will return delighted and must tell you of the interesting evening classes she is now attending. The alcoholic, who used to get herself into trouble each month, will discuss the dream holiday she is planning. The husband comes to tell you about his wife 'who is now the woman I married'. There is the mother who is so delighted because 'even the children are behaving nowadays' and the student who has happily passed her final examinations, the epileptic mother whose children are once more returned home to her care and the asthmatic who drove to London Bridge ceremonially to throw overboard her now redundant aerosol inhalers. For women, who have suffered some of the serious consequences of the premenstrual syndrome that we have discussed in earlier chapters, it is really no hardship to have to administer their progesterone by pessary, suppository or injection, instead of the more conventional way through the mouth.

Progesterone Suppositories

The progesterone suppositories are small pellets of inert wax containing progesterone. The wax melts at body temperature releasing the progesterone which is absorbed through the lining of the vagina or rectum and conveyed in the blood to where it is needed. The wax is expelled from the body either moistening the vagina or mixed with the faeces.

Women who have vaginal infections are invariably treated with pessaries and there are rarely any complaints. Suppositories, too, are easy enough to insert into the anus. Suppositories were used by the ancient Egyptians, Greeks and Romans for the administration of drugs to the rectum, where they are easily absorbed into the bloodstream, but they have never been a popular method of treatment in Britain.

During a recent holiday in Spain we were enjoying a pleasant evening with our Spanish hosts when their four-year-old daughter emerged into the lounge complaining she couldn't go to sleep because of earache. The mother searched in her handbag, gave the little one a suppository which she took away and apparently used herself quite satisfactorily. Women who have learnt to appreciate the value of progesterone no longer object to using pessaries or suppositories.

Many years of research preceded the introduction of commercially produced progesterone suppositories. The base in which the progesterone was dissolved had to be carefully selected, as the original ones tended to cause irritation and diarrhoea. Regulation of the temperature appeared important while preparing the suppositories to prevent the formation of crystals, which produced a painful pin-pricking sensation when inserted. If the suppository melted at too high a temperature, those women with low body temperatures complained of grittiness.

In practice, progesterone suppositories and pessaries are interchangeable and it is usually left to the individual which route she uses, or she can use both on alternate occasions. Patients are given permission to use an extra suppository or pessary when an unexpected need arises, such as when a sudden surge of irritability is building up or an impending migraine threatens. Up to six 400 mg. suppositories can be used in a day. After all, during pregnancy the blood level of progesterone is so high that it would need thirty suppositories daily to reach that level. If two suppositories are used simultaneously in the same orifice the melted wax prevents further absorption of progesterone, so it is impossible for an individual to overdose with this method. It is important to advise women not to insert a tampon at the same time as a pessary, otherwise the tampon absorbs the progesterone and she receives no benefit.

The time of giving progesterone will be determined by observing each individual patient's chart. In the normal case it is given as suppositories or pessaries from ovulation until the onset of menstruation. However, if symptoms continue until the second or third day of menstruation then the progesterone should be continued until the fourth day. If symptoms start at ovulation the progesterone should be started a couple of days beforehand. In short there should be individual tailoring for each patient. The progesterone needs to be started at ovulation, or at least four days before the symptoms would be expected, and continued until menstruation has started. Therefore it is quite useless to give suppositories on alternate days from day 19 to 25. This was how it was used in the double blind controlled trial reported by Smith, which is often quoted to claim that progesterone is ineffective because it was unsuccessful in that particular trial. The progesterone could never have demonstrated its effectiveness as it was used too late, without regard for the individual variation in the length of cycle, for too short a time and with too long an interval between the administration of progesterone.

There is a marked variation in the absorption of progesterone by individuals. Some absorb it quickly and others more slowly, some show immediate increase in the blood progesterone level, while in others the rise or fall is slower. Furthermore, there is a small proportion of women, between 5% and 10%, who do not absorb progesterone effectively from the rectum or vagina, and who will need it to be given by injection. The absorption of pessaries and suppositories is usually quick and within twenty minutes there may be a rise in the level of progesterone in the blood, but the progesterone level may drop quite quickly too, and the rise is always over within twenty-four hours while in some women

the effect only lasts four hours. This means that most women
need to take at least two daily, some even need six.

Progesterone Injections

Progesterone injections last longer. In some women they
only need to be repeated on alternate days, while others
need them daily. The absorption is more reliable with injections and so they are used in desperate situations, such as
when a marriage is at breaking point, or children are in
danger of being taken into care. Another advantage is that
if the injection is given daily by a district nurse, she can
silently supervise those who need watching in the premenstruum, for instance where there is risk of suicide, battering
or an alcoholic bout. Injections are more convenient for
patients in hospitals and are also used where suppositories
and pessaries have failed.

At first the injections are given by the practice, district or
factory nurse, but with suitable instruction most patients
soon learn the art of giving their own injections. Failing this
the husband may be ready to learn the technique. In the
buttocks between the muscles fibres there are clumps of fat
cells which form a cushion for us to sit on. The progesterone
injection should be inserted into the buttock muscles, where
it is absorbed by the fat cells and then gradually released into
the blood. The injections should not be given into the thigh
or arm, where there are no fat cells between the muscle
fibres. The injection can be given anywhere in the buttocks
where there is a one-inch pinch of flesh, which means it
cannot be given in the upper inner quadrant, where the skin
is closely attached to the end of the spine.

Progesterone Implant

Progesterone can also be given by implants to those who
have already had complete relief of symptoms with either
pessaries, suppositories or injections, as it relieves the need
for daily medication and lasts for an average of three or four

months and occasionally for as long as eighteen months. It is particularly useful for women who have had their womb removed, as they will not be troubled by the erratic menstruation which sometimes occurs. It is also used for those who are forgetful in giving themselves progesterone, such as the feckless alcoholics. One patient living in Italy calculated that the cost of an annual implant, plus the air fare from Rome, was cheaper than the cost of daily suppositories.

However, a progesterone implant is not as convenient as an oestrogen implant. More progesterone pellets are used and they sometimes have a tendency to be extruded, or pushed out. Attempts at extrusion are likely to occur at times of greatest progesterone need, such as during the premenstruum. The site of the implant may become inflamed but it can be eased by giving progesterone injections for five consecutive days, thus temporarily giving the body an alternative supply of progesterone.

A progesterone implant should not be given to those hoping to conceive within twelve months; those unduly concerned when their normal menstruation is replaced by an irregular scanty loss or possibly missed menstruation for spells of six months; those who must avoid premenstrual symptoms at all costs, such as the epileptic woman who may not appreciate her implanted supply of progesterone is running low and has an epileptic attack at a most unfortunate and potentially dangerous time; and those whose normal daily requirement of progesterone is very high.

If progesterone is given daily by pessaries, suppositories or injections and then stopped for some reason, menstruation will occur. This is similar to what happens when the level of progesterone drops and menstruation occurs in a normal cycle.

It is impossible to give an overdose of progesterone to a woman who has borne children, because during pregnancy women are exposed to a thirtyfold increase in their blood progesterone level for nine full months, instead of just a mere two weeks, and the body has learnt to deal with that. On the other hand in childless and immature women an excess of progesterone may very occasionally cause euphoria and restless energy, insomnia and dysmenorrhoea or uterine cramps similar to those suffered in spasmodic dysmenorrhoea.

There are no contra-indications when progesterone cannot be used. Also there are no risks of progesterone producing cancer; indeed, progesterone is used in the treatment of some cancers, especially those produced in the vagina of teenage girls who were exposed to stilboestrol (DES) during their foetal life, and also in advanced or recurrent cancer of the womb. If there is any possibility of thrush or yeast infection being present, this should be cleared up before pessaries are used, as progesterone may encourage the thrush to grow. It is also necessary to treat the partner with antifungal tablets to ensure that he does not reinfect the patient.

Progesterone suppositories in doses of 200 mg. and 400 mg. are commercially available in Britain under the trade name of 'Cyclogest', distributed and marketed by Hoechst UK Ltd, Pharmaceutical Division, Hoechst House, Salisbury Road, Hounslow, Middlesex.

Progestogens

Because of the difficulty that progesterone cannot be given by mouth, the biochemists sought for a synthetic preparation which could be absorbed orally. They tried making small alterations to the chemical formulae of progesterone hoping to find one with slightly different properties. After all, the formulae of oestrogen, testosterone and cortisone are all very similar, although they have quite different properties. The biochemists succeeded in finding the progestogens, which are the basis of all the contraceptive pills and gave rise to a multi-million-pound industry. When the progestogens were first discovered it was believed that they were true progesterone substitutes but in effect they have some properties of oestrogen, some of progesterone, and some of testosterone. If progestogens have been given during pregnancy and the child is a girl, she is likely to show masculinizing effects in her genitals and be a tomboy with marked aggression. This is quite different from the effect of natural progesterone which is produced in such large quantities during pregnancy. Indeed, surveys have suggested that if progesterone is given to mothers before the sixteenth week of pregnancy for eight weeks or longer, the child of that pregnancy has a tendency towards an enhanced intelligence, with a good academic record, more examination passes and a better chance of reaching university than control children whose mothers did not have progesterone.

There are many differences between progesterone and the various progestogens, but unfortunately there are still some doctors who do not realize this. Progesterone lowers the blood pressure while progestogens raise it, and whereas progesterone raises SHBG levels, progestogens lower it. Progestogens are not used by progesterone receptors. Progesterone can relieve water and sodium retention whereas some progestogens, such as norethisterone used in the pill, cause retention of water and sodium. Progesterone is converted by the adrenals into all the other steroids, such as cortisone, oestrogen and testosterone, which is not possible with the progestogens. The function of progesterone is also to maintain a pregnancy and it is now used in increasing amounts in invitro fertilisation, but the progestogens cannot be used for this purpose. Some progestogens have an oestrogenic effect as well, which is useful in the contraceptive field. Disposal of progestogens from the body differs from that of natural progesterone, which is excreted in the urine or faeces as pregnanediol.

The usual progestogens in the pill cause a lowering of the blood progesterone level (see Fig. 34), and this is why women with premenstrual symptoms so often have difficulty in tolerating the pill whether it is the oestrogen-progestogen or the progestogen-only pill or tolerating the progestogen tablets in menopausal preparations.

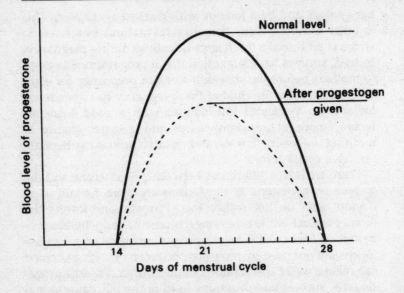

Fig. 34 Effect of progestogen on the blood level of progesterone

Contraception

For those who have, or have had, spasmodic dysmenorrhoea the oestrogen-progestogen pill is usually the best method of contraception. These women have a low oestrogen level and benefit when given some extra oestrogen; in fact many of these women were sorry when the high oestrogen pills were removed from the market, as they said they felt so much better on a high dose. On the other hand premenstrual syndrome sufferers are those who tend to have difficulty with the pill, causing an increase in headaches, gain in weight, depression and nausea, and these women are candidates for the more serious blood-clotting problems. Furthermore the progestogens tend to lower the normal progesterone level, making their premenstrual syndrome worse.

Unfortunately the intra-uterine devices have a tendency, in some women, to make menstruation heavier or longer, and therefore are best avoided in those who already have heavy periods. They should also be avoided by those who have previously had pelvic inflammatory disease.

Women who are having progesterone treatment for premenstrual syndrome can either take a progestogen-only pill from day 1 until day 13 and then start the normal progesterone dose until menstruation, or they can start with a small amount of progesterone from day 8, say half a 200 mg. progesterone suppository, until their normal course of progesterone at ovulation, which they will continue up to the start of menstruation. In this way they are contraceptively safe. Progesterone is Nature's natural contraceptive; it is present after ovulation and converts the thin mucus into a thick sticky type in which sperms cannot enter the womb.

Sterilization
Sterilization is not the ultimate universal answer to contraception, for women with premenstrual syndrome may find the operation increases their symptoms (see page 31). Recently, Dr B. W. McGuiness, a family practitioner in Cheshire, England, in a controlled series found that women who have bilateral tubal ligation suffered significantly more menstrual cycle disturbances post-operatively. His findings have since been confirmed by others.

Conception
Those women on progesterone treatment who are anxious to conceive, are advised to start their progesterone 48 hours after the temperature chart shows ovulation has occurred, or if they do not know when ovulation occurs they should start on day 16 for cycles up to 28 days, and on day 18 for longer cycles. They should be advised to continue the progesterone until the pregnancy is confirmed and then only stop if they are free from pregnancy symptoms.

Testosterone

Testosterone, the male hormone, has in the past been occasionally used for the treatment of premenstrual syndrome, especially in those who have sore breasts premenstrually. It is effective, especially in giving energy, and lightening or stopping menstruation, and easing the engorged breasts. However, it can have masculinizing effects, such as hoarseness, a deepening of the voice, and the growing of hair on the beard area of the face. Testosterone is also valuable in rapidly stopping menopausal flushes and depression when it is given in a combined tablet with oestrogen. Testosterone also improves the sex urge and activity, and may be used in implants together with oestrogen.

Bromocriptine

Bromocriptine is capable of lowering a raised prolactin level. As explained in Chapter 18 sometimes a raised prolactin level interferes with the progesterone feedback pathway from the womb to the hypothalamus. There are reports from Holland that patients with infertility and premenstrual syndrome have been successfully treated with bromocriptine. However, double blind trials on patients in England carried out by Ghose and Coppen, using a different dose, have not confirmed these findings. Patients who appear to benefit from bromocriptine are those with a raised prolactin level and marked water retention, painful and engorged breasts, those who have lost their sex interest and those who have recently had a postnatal depression.

Pyridoxine

Pyridoxine, or vitamin B6, has been recommended for women who become depressed when using oestrogen-progestogen contraception, and for menopausal women receiving oestrogen replacement therapy. Unfortunately worldwide clinical trials have failed to show the value of pyridoxine in women with well-diagnosed premenstrual syndrome. The recommended daily requirement of B6 is only 2–4 mg., yet doses of ten or even a hundred times that amount are often prescribed. Schaumberg, an American neurologist, had the task of giving animals peripheral neuritis so that a possible curative drug might be developed. Peripheral neuritis is a painful, chronic, debilitating disease occurring commonly in diabetics and alcoholics. The animals were given vitamin B6 (pyridoxine) and the team of which he was a member reported that pyridoxine overdose could cause degeneration of the peripheral sensory neurones (nerve endings) in the dog and rat. In 1983 Schaumberg and his colleagues reported peripheral neuropathy resulting from massive pyridoxine overdose in five women and two men, who had similar degeneration of their peripheral sensory neurones revealed at biopsy. In my practice, with my son, Dr Michael Dalton, we tested all women currently taking pyridoxine, and of the 172 women whose blood pyridoxine level was above the normal range it was noted that 60% had neurological symptoms. The symptoms of pyridoxine overdose include pins and needles particularly of the hands and feet; areas of numbness sometimes around the mouth or on the limbs; oversensitivity of the skin with itching and crawling sensations; as well as muscle weakness, with difficulty typing, playing the piano, running, climbing stairs, until finally a walking stick or wheelchair is needed (see Fig. 35). The study showed no difference in the incidence of neurological symptoms with the dose of pyridoxine currently being taken, which varied from 25 mg. to 500 mg. daily. However, there was a difference as far as length of time that pyridoxine had been taken, irrespective of whether it was taken daily or intermittently, neurological symptoms appeared after six months. It does not matter whether pyridoxine is taken alone, with other B vitamins, with other vitamins or with magnesium – the incidence of symptoms of overdose is the same. Fortunately when pyridoxine is abruptly stopped there are no withdrawal symptoms, no further progression and a gradual recovery from the temporary disabilities.

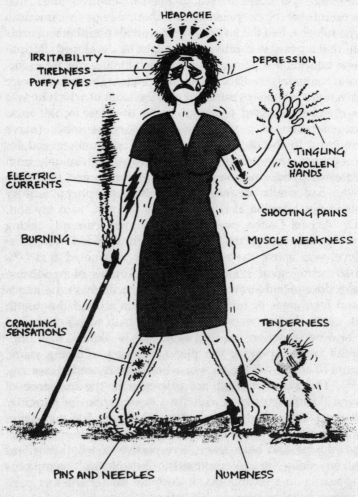

HEADACHE

IRRITABILITY
TIREDNESS
PUFFY EYES

DEPRESSION

TINGLING
SWOLLEN
HANDS

ELECTRIC
CURRENTS

SHOOTING PAINS

BURNING

MUSCLE WEAKNESS

CRAWLING
SENSATIONS

TENDERNESS

PINS AND NEEDLES   NUMBNESS

Fig. 35 Symptoms of B6 overdose

Clonidine

Clonidine is a drug for the lowering of blood pressure, and in very small doses is marketed under the name of 'Dixarit', when it may be used to relieve menopausal flushes in those who for some reason are unable to tolerate oestrogens. However, it only acts on the flushes and is of no value in relieving the other oestrogen-deficiency symptoms at the menopause, such as vagina and skin thinning, joint pains and the psychological symptoms. One beautiful menopausal lady, who always had a perfectly coiffured head of white hair, refused to have a further course of oestrogens, which although they cured her menopausal flushes and depression, caused some of her white hairs to become grey again. She opted for clonidine, at least for a few months until the psychological symptoms bore down on her.

Diuretics

It is best to avoid diuretics as any help they give to those with water retention is only temporary, and it is so easy to repeat them indefinitely, always taking more and more until the balance of sodium and potassium is disturbed. Diuretics do not help premenstrual tension, depression or irritability, only symptoms due to water retention, such as bloatedness, gain in weight and swollen ankles. Once addicted to diuretics it is difficult to come off and this must be done gradually, reducing from four to three, then three to two at monthly intervals, always reducing in the postmenstruum. When the dose is down to one daily, the reduction should be to alternate days, then every third day and every fourth day, before finally stopping in the postmenstruum.

Potassium

A lowering of the blood potassium level may be suspected in those who have been taking diuretics for a long time, those who have food cravings and prolonged dieting and those who complain of exhaustion and muscle weakness throughout the cycle. These women should have a blood potassium estimation, and if a low level is found they should take potassium tablets until the deficiency is corrected and change to a potassium sparing diuretic.

22

A Fairer Future

This book was written with the aim of spreading the news to mankind that the once-a-month miseries of countless women can be, and are being, successfully relieved and treated. At the same time it was hoped that it would help men to understand and appreciate the menstrual problems of women and become partners in helping them through those difficult days. That you are reading this brings hope that the aim will be achieved.

The menstrual miseries are widespread and incapacitating at times; their effects can involve all classes and all ages of both sexes. Nevertheless it is possible to abolish dysmenorrhoea, premenstrual syndrome and menopausal problems by hormone treatment. But although treatment is possible it is not yet universal. Menopausal clinics are now well established and are countrywide, and gynaecological help is available for the relief of symptoms related to the change of life. The recognition of premenstrual syndrome is not yet as widespread, although since the first edition of this book there have been some encouraging signs. Well Women Clinics, funded by voluntary contributions, are being developed throughout Britain with the aim of treating premenstrual syndrome and menstrual problems, as well as to enable the early detection of cancer of the breast and cervix. The Family Planning Association now accepts responsibility for education and help in menstrual and sexual problems, which includes premenstrual syndrome. Even if the nearest FPA Clinic cannot help, the local headquarters are usually helpful in advising where women can best obtain help locally.

Premenstrual syndrome really should be a speciality of general practice, and should be mastered by every general practitioner. Ever-increasing numbers of general practitioners and consultants are now able to diagnose, treat and manage all cases of premenstrual syndrome which come within their orbit. The long-term follow-up of a chronic disease such as premenstrual syndrome is best done by a general practitioner, the physician of continuing care, rather than in the hospitals, with their ever-changing junior staff and their need to discharge patients as soon as possible to make way for the new ones.

The gynaecologist tends to be satisfied with a faultless physical examination and the reassurance of a 'D&C' and is then content to refer the patient back to the family doctor. The endocrinologists have more serious diseases to occupy their time and rarely wish to be troubled by disturbances of menstrual hormones, especially at a time when there are not enough useful hormonal estimations to clinch the diagnosis and determine the dose of hormones needed. Psychiatrists do occasionally recognize the syndrome, prescribe anti-depressants or tranquillizers, but then see the patient in her symptom-free postmenstruum and discharge her from their care. The neurologists fully investigate all cases of epilepsy and migraine to satisfy themselves that no lesion is present and discharge the patient. The chest physician treats the asthma, the rhinologist the allergic rhinitis, the orthopaedic surgeon and rheumatologist the backache and painful joints, the dermatologists the herpes and neurodermatitis, but even if all the menstrually related symptoms are appreciated by these consultants, the diagnosis is still too easily ignored.

One dream was short lived. The University of Oklahoma for a short while in 1989–90 led the world in having a Department of Premenstrual Syndrome with a multidisciplinary staff working together to bring relief to sufferers of premenstrual syndrome. They were responsible for the conducting of clinics for the diagnosis and treatment of premenstrual syndrome, teaching medical students, residents and other professionals, and organizing research aimed at helping women worldwide. It is hoped that by the time the next edition of this book is needed other universities in other countries, and especially in Britain, will appreciate the need for a permanent, not temporary, department for work on premenstrual syndrome.

If Premenstrual Syndrome Clinics are to be established the general practitioner will need to be in the forefront, assisted by a psychiatrist and gynaecologist, for it is only the general practitioner who encompasses the whole vista of symptoms and knows the effect on the family. Before he is ready to accept this role the general practitioner needs specialized courses in diagnosing and treating these menstrual problems, and medical students require a greater familiarity with the subject during their undergraduate training. The general practitioner needs to know the art of adjusting menstruation for vital events, knowing the hazards and methods, the utilization of the peak postmenstrual days and recognizing the women with dysmenorrhoea and premenstrual syndrome who urgently need treatment. A nurse or trained person can instruct patients in keeping a menstrual chart and supervise their three-hourly starch eating pattern.

The National Commission for Women in 1985 recommended to the Cabinet the need for greater undergraduate and postgraduate education on premenstrual syndrome and the need for training teachers, social workers, police and lawyers to better understand the problem.

The need for greater public education and awareness is obvious, and here is an opportunity to be grasped by the media and offered to a public always hungry for human stories of medical possibilities, but we must remember that doctors do not like to be told by the popular press what treatment they should give their patients. Education on these subjects is already included in the GCSE syllabus so it is hoped that both the women and men of tomorrow will have a greater appreciation of these problems and the solutions which are to hand. In the 1989 Midland Examination Board the question was asked, 'What do the letters "PMT" stand for?'

It is estimated that the cost of menstrual problems to British industry is equal to 3% of the total wage bill. Would it not be better for British industry to invest a fraction of that sum in Menstrual Clinics and training schemes for doctors, in order to speed the time when such wastage can be eliminated?

School and university examinations can be made fairer by adjusting the timetable so that papers are set a week apart, by having compulsory questions in both papers rather than one compulsory paper, by setting alternative dates where possible, and making available a choice of dates for practical and oral examinations. Where practical, teachers can set pupils' work two or more weeks in advance. The GCSE has done much to improve the lot of the premenstrual syndrome candidate, who can now present the project work she carried out in her postmenstrual peak.

A greater appreciation of the relationship of the premenstrual syndrome to violence and battering would enable premenstrual baby-battering to be correctly diagnosed, understood and treated, so eliminating the problem and removing the social stigmas of separation, children being taken into care, and criminal proceedings.

The ideal would seem to be to abolish menstruation altogether at those times when conception is not required. This is possible by the prolonged administration of progestogens, but not yet ideal. Initially there tends to be the occasional breakthrough bleeding, and then after a year or two there is a subtle change in the personality of the woman: she becomes harder, more efficient and loses interest in sex. Is the price worth it? Already there is the technique of menstrual aspiration which women can learn to perform on themselves, in which they suck the menstrual flow from the womb through a thin flexible plastic tube and complete menstruation in one minute or less. Unfortunately menstrual hormones may be upset by this event and their smooth ebb and flow drastically altered. The layman, or rather laywoman, too eagerly hopes that the mere removal of the womb will accomplish the feat, but as has already been discussed the removal of the womb too often upsets the hormonal pathway and the end result may be worse than before the operation.

In the last century John Ruskin reminded his fellow countrymen that 'the true wealth of the Nation was running to waste' because most children had no sort of education. The same could be said today about the lack of education and understanding of premenstrual syndrome. The discussion of menstruation and its attendant problems should be as open and unrestricted as the discussion of sex, for the knowledge and understanding of menstruation should be available to all.

Having read as far as this, there will probably be two questions nagging at your mind. 'If progesterone and oestrogen are so successful in their respective treatments, why are more doctors not using them?' and 'Why do some doctors prefer to use a drug which is less successful and only brings partial relief to a portion of patients with mild symptoms, rather than one which brings complete relief to most patients with mild and severe symptoms?'

There is no simple answer to these perfectly reasonable questions. Some answers are contained in earlier chapters, but there are a number of other reasons which can be roughly grouped under three broad headings:

- 1 Doctors have an essentially conservative approach.
- 2 Commercial aspects.
- 3 Lack of consultancy and treatment facilities.

Very few of the doctors in practice today had any training in diagnosing or treating what we now know is the world's commonest disease, premenstrual syndrome. Nor have they received much training in nutrition and it is rare for them to ask a patient for a detailed account of her day's diet. It is easy enough to plead there is no time to take a dietary history, but this can just as easily be left for the nurse to prepare and show to the doctor. Doctors are themselves wholly responsible for the diagnosis and treatment of their patients and they alone have the right to decide what treatment they believe is best. They have to protect their patients as well as themselves, and therefore have a natural reticence about using treatments which they personally are not yet fully persuaded are safe and effective. However, this does place on them the responsibility for increasing their knowledge of the subject, for the average British general practitioner will have in his practice some 50 women with premenstrual syndrome needing treatment.

The general practitioner, who has a patient with a condition he does not understand, will forward that patient to a consultant who specializes in that particular problem. But to whom will he send the premenstrual asthma or the premenstrual sinusitis which has been confirmed by a menstrual chart? Not to a gynaecologist or endocrinologist or psychiatrist.

These are but partial answers to these questions, but it must be appreciated that the number of doctors who can diagnose and treat these menstrual problems increases month by month. If more clinics could be established and training courses instituted the number of undiagnosed and untreated sufferers would steadily decrease.

In 1986 the Dalton Society, an international medical society, was founded with the object of furthering knowledge and research into premenstrual syndrome. They have held symposiums in Los Angeles, Chicago, Tulsa and Oklahoma City, attended by doctors from all over the world, where research papers were read and discussions held on improvement in treatment and better understanding of the causes. There are also 'friends of the society' who, although not in the medical field, are anxious to contribute funds and their energy to the alleviation of the problems brought on by premenstrual syndrome – surely a worthwhile charity, deserving of generous support.

A quotation by Henry David Thoreau runs:

You are building castles in the air!
And that is right, that is where they should be.
What we have to do is put the foundations under them.

Let us get down to work.

Useful Addresses

PMS Help
Po Box 160
St Albans
Hertfordshire AL1 4UQ

National Childbirth Trust
9 Queensborough Terrace
London W2
tel: 071–221 3833

The Hysterectomy Society
c/o Mrs J Vaughan
Rivendell
Warren Way
Lower Heswall
Wirral
Merseyside
tel: 051 342 3167

Association for Postnatal
Illness
25 Jerdan Place
Fulham
London SW6 1BE
tel: 071–731 4867

Meet-A-Mum-Association
[MAMA]
26a Cumnor Hill
Oxford OX2 9HA

Relaxation for Living
"Dunesk"
29 Burwood Park Road
Walton-on-Thames
Surrey KT12 5LH
tel: 0932 227826

Endometriosis Society
65 Holmdene Avenue
Herne Hill
London SE24
tel: 071–737 4764

Aramant Trust
16–24 Lonsdale Road
London NW6 6RD

National Osteoporosis
Society
Po Box 10
Radstock
Bath
Avon BA3 3YB

Dalton Society
℅ 41 Harlesden Road
St Albans
Hertfordshire AL1 4LE

Other Publications by the Author

'The Premenstrual Syndrome' (1953) (Joint authorship with R. Greene) *British Medical Journal*, I, 1007.

The Similarity of Symptomatology of Premenstrual Syndrome and Toxaemia of Pregnancy and their Response to Progesterone' (1954) BMA Prize Essay, *British Medical Journal*, II, 1071.

'Discussion on the Premenstrual Syndrome' (1955) *Proceedings of the Royal Society of Medicine*, 48, 5, 337–47 (Section of General Practice 5–15).

'Progesterone in Toxaemia of Pregnancy' (1955) *Medical World*.

'The Aftermath of Hysterectomy and Oopherectomy' (1957) *Proc. Roy. Soc. Med.*, 50, 6, 415–18 (Section of General Practice, p. 13–16)

'Toxaemia of Pregnancy Treated with Progesterone during the Symptomatic Stage' (1957) *BMJ*, II, 378–81.

'Menstruation and Acute Psychiatric Illnesses' (1959) *BMJ*, I, 148–9.

'Menstrual Disorders in General Practice' (1959) *Journal of the Royal College of General Practitioners*, 2, 236.

'Comparative Trials of New Oral Progestogenic Compounds in Treatment of Premenstrual Syndrome' (1959) *BMJ*, II, 1307–09.

'Early Symptoms of Pre-Eclamptic Toxaemia' (1960) *The Lancet*, p. 198–199.

'Effect of Menstruation on Schoolgirls' Weekly Work' (1960) *BMJ*, I, 326–8.

'Menstruation and Accidents' (1960) *BMJ*, II, 1425–26.

'Schoolgirls' Behaviour and Menstruation' *BMJ*, II, 1647–49.

'Menstruation and Crime' (1961) *BMJ*, II, 1752–53.

'Controlled Trials in the Prophylactic Value of Progesterone in the Treatment of Pre-Eclamptic Toxaemia' (1962) *Journal of Obstetrics and Gynaecology of the British Commonwealth*, LXIX, 3, 463–68.

'The Present Position of Progestational Steroids in the Treatment of Premenstrual Syndrome' (1963) *Medical Women's Federation Journal*, 137–140.

'Notes on the Use of the Menstrual Chart' (1964) *Drug and Therapeutics Bulletin*.

'The Influence of Mother's Menstruation on her Child' (1966) *Proc. Roy. Soc. Med.*, 59, 10, 1014–16, (Section of General Practice with Section of Paediatrics), BMA Prize Essay.

'Influence of Menstruation on Glaucoma' (1967) *British Journal of Ophthalmology*, 51, 10, 692–95. BMA Prize.

'Ante-Natal Progesterone and Intelligence' (1968) *British Journal of Psychiatry*, 114, 1377–82.

'Menstruation and Examinations' (1968) *The Lancet*, 1386–88.

'Children's Hospital Admissions and Mother's Menstruation' (1970) *BMJ*, II, 27–28.

'The Importance of Menstrual Dates' (1970) *Update*, 310–14.

'Prospective Study into Puerperal Depression' (1971) *British Journal of Psychiatry*, 118, 547, 689–92.

'Puerperal and Premenstrual Depression' (1971) *Proc. Roy. Soc. Med.* 64, 12, 1249–52, (Section of General Practice 43–4)

'Ovulation Symptoms and Avoidance of Conception' (1972) *The Lancet*, 437–38.

'The General Practitioner and Research' (1973) *The Practitioner*, 210, 784–88.

'Progesterone Suppositories and Pessaries in the Treatment of Menstrual Migraine' (1973) *Headache*, 12, 4, 151–9.

'Premenstrual Ankle Edema in Young Girl' (1974) *Journal of American Medical Association*, 228.

'Migraine in General Practice' (1973) *Journal of the Royal College of General Practitioners*, 23, 97–106, Migraine Trust Prize Essay 1972.

'Do it Yourself' (1975) British Migraine Association, Migraine Newsletter.

'The Effect of Progesterone on Brain Function' (1975) Proceedings of the Acta Endocrin Congress, Amsterdam.

'Postpubertal Effects of Prenatal Administration of Progesterone' (1975) Society for Research in Child Development.

'The Influence of Menstruation' (1973) *Update*, 883–39.

'Premenstrual Syndrome' (1975) *Update*, 121–8.

'Food Intake prior to a Migraine Attack – Study of 2313 Spontaneous Attacks' (1975) *Headache*, 15, 3, 188–93.

'Migraine and Oral Contraceptives' (1976) *Headache*, 15, 4, 247–51.

'Prenatal Progesterone and Educational Attainments' (1976) *British Journal of Psychiatry*, 129, 438–42, The Charles Oliver Hawthorne BMA Prize Essay 1976.

'A Clinician's View' (1976) *Royal Society of Health Journal*.

'Menstruation and Sport' (1976) chapter in *Sports Medicine* 2nd edition. ed. J. P. R. Williams and P. N. Sperryn, (Edward Arnold, London).

'Treatment of the Premenstrual Syndrome' (1976) *Journal of Pharmacotherapy*, 51–55.

'Bromocriptine and Premenstrual Syndrome' (1976) *Pharmacological and Clinical Aspects of Bromocriptine*, ed. R. I. Bayliss, P. Turner and W. P. McClay, MSC Consultants, London.

'Premenstrual Syndrome with Psychiatric Symptoms' (1977) *Journal of the American Medical Association*, 238, 25, 2729.

'Synthetic Progestins vs Natural Generic Progesterone: Pharmacologic Properties' (1978) *Journal of the American Medical Association*, 240, 6.

'Menarcheal Age in the Disabled' (1978) *BMJ*, 2, 475, joint authorship with Maureen E. Dalton.

'Intelligence and Prenatal Progesterone: A Reappraisal' (1979) *Journal of the Royal Society of Medicine*, 72, 397–99.

'Food Intake Before Migraine Attacks in Children' (1979) *Journal of the Royal College of General Practitioners*, 29, 662–5, joint authorship with Maureen E. Dalton.

'Intelligence and Prenatal Progesterone' (1979) *Journal of the Royal Society of Medicine*, 72, 951.

'Cyclic Posthysterectomy Symptoms' (1980) *Journal of the American Medicine Association*, 244, 13, 1497.

'Cyclical Criminal Acts in Premenstrual Syndrome' (1980) *The Lancet*, 1070–71.

'The Effect of Progesterone and Progestogens on the Foetus' (1981) *Neuropharmacology*.

'Violence and the Premenstrual Syndrome' (1981) *Journal of Police Surgeons of Great Britain*.

'Legal Implications of Premenstrual Syndrome' (1972) *World Medicine*.

'Overview of Premenstrual Syndrome' (1982) chapter in *Behaviour and the Menstrual Cycle*, ed. R. Friedman, (Marchel and Dekker, New York).

'Premenstrual Syndrome and its Treatment' (1982) *International Medicine*, 2, 2, 10–13.

'What is this PMS?' (1982) *Journal of the Royal College of General Practice*, 717–19.

'Pyridoxine Overdose in Premenstrual Syndrome' (1985) *The Lancet*, 1168.

'Progesterone Prophylaxis Used Successfully in Postnatal Depression' (1985) *The Practitioner*, 229, 507.

'Premenstrual Syndrome: A New Criminal Defence?' (1983) co-author with Lawrence Taylor, *California Western Law Review*, 18, 2, 268–86.

'The Depression of PMS and Menstrual Distress' (1984) *Mimms Magazine*, March 1984, 32–37.

'Menstruation and Migraine' (1984) *Migraine Matters*, 2, 1, 6–8.

'Diagnosis and Clinical Feature of Premenstrual Syndrome' (1984) chapter in *Premenstrual Syndrome and Dysmenorrhoeoa* ed. M. Y. Dawood, (Urban and Schwarzburg).

'Erythema Multiforme Associated with Menstruation' (1985) *Journal of the Royal Society of Medicine*, 78, 787, Sept. 1985.

'Menstrual Stress' (1985) Stress Medicine, 1, 127–133.

'Vitamins: A New Perspective' (1986) *Mimms Magazine*, March 1986.

'Premenstrual Syndrome' (1986) *Hamline Law Review*, 9, 1, 143–154, Spring.

'Should Premenstrual Syndrome be a Legal Defence' (1986) chapter in *Premenstrual Syndrome: Ethical implications in a Bio-Behavioural Perspective*, ed. B. F. Carter and B. E. Ginsburg.

'Nasal Absorption of Progesterone in Women' (1987) *Brit. J. Ob. and Gynaec.*, January 1987, 94, 84–88. Co-author with M. E. Dalton, D. R. Bromham, C. L. Ambrose and J. Osborne.

'The Efficacy of Progesterone Suppositories as a Contraception in Women with Severe PMS' (1987) co-author M. E. Dalton, and K. Guthrie, *British Journal of Family Planning*, 13, 87–89.

'Premenstrual Syndrome and Thyroid' (1987) Accepted by *Integrative Psychiatry*.

'Characteristics of Pyridoxine Overdose Neuropathy Syndrome' (1987) co-author with M. J. T. Dalton, *Acta Neurologica Scandinavica*, 76, 8–11. Awarded Cullen Prize.

'What is this PMS?' (1987) chapter in *The Psychology of Women – Ongoing Debates* ed. Mary Roth Walsh, (Yale University Press).

'Incidence of PMS in Twins' (1987) co-author M. E. Dalton and K. Guthrie, *BMJ*, 295, 1027–28.

'Trial of Progesterone Vaginal Suppositories in the Treatment of Premenstrual Syndrome' (1987) letter in *Am. J. Obstet. Gynecol.*, 156, 6, 1555

'Premenstrual Syndrome & Thyroid Dysfunction' (1987) *Integr. Psychiatry*, 5, 179–93.

'Treating the Premenstrual Syndrome' (1988) *BMJ*, 297, 490.

'Progesterone for Premenstrual Exacerbations of Asthma' (1988) *The Lancet*, 8912, 684.

'Successful Prophylactic Progesterone for Idiopathic Postnatal Depression' (1989) *International Journal of Prenatal & Perinatal Studies*, 323–27.

'Hypothesis: The Aetiology of Premenstrual Syndrome is with the Progesterone Receptors' (1990) *Medical Hypothesis 1990*, May.

'Postpartum Depression & Bonding' (1989) *Int. J. Prenatal & Perinatal Studies 1989*, 225–26.

'Do Progesterone Receptors Have a Role in PMS?' (1990) accepted for publication *Int. J. Prenatal & Perinatal Studies*.

Premenstrual Syndrome (1964) (Heinemann Medical Books, London).

The Menstrual Cycle (1969) (Penguin Books, London and Pantheon Books, Random House, New York).

Premenstrual Syndrome and Progesterone Therapy (1977)

(Heinemann Medical Books, London and Year Book Inc., Chicago).

Depression After Childbirth (1980) (Oxford University Press, Oxford). Revised 2nd Edition published January 1989.

Premenstrual Syndrome and Progesterone Therapy (1984) (Heinemann Medical Books, London and Year Book Inc., Chicago). Revised 2nd edition.

PMS Illustrated (1990) (Peter Andrew Publishing Co.)

PMS in Court (1990) (Peter Andrew Publishing Co.)

Glossary

Abortion	death of foetus
Adrenal glands	two glands situated above the kidneys and responsible for producing numerous hormones
Adrenalin	one of the hormones produced by the adrenal glands
Amenorrhoea	absence of menstruation
Analgesic	drug taken to relieve pain
Anovular	without ovulation
Anorexia	loss of appetite
Antenatal	before childbirth
Antidepressant	drug to remove depression
Anus	exit from the alimentary canal, or back passage
Bromocriptine	a drug which lowers the prolactin level
Cervical smear	test for the diagnosis of cancer of the neck of the womb
Climacteric	change of life
Corticosteroids	hormones produced in the cortex of the adrenal glands
Diuretics	drugs capable of increasing the amount of urine passed

Dysmenorrhoea	pain with periods
Dyspareunia	pain on intercourse
Embyro	developing ovum up to end of eighth week after conception
Endocrine gland	organ releasing hormones into the blood to act on distant cells
Endocrinologist	one who studies the effects of the endocrine glands
Endometrium	inner lining of the womb
Fallopian tubes	two tubes leading from the ovaries to the womb along which the egg cells pass.
Foetus	developing human from the third month of pregnancy until birth
Follicle stimulating hormone	hormone produced by the pituitary acting on the ovary to ripen the follicles and produce oestrogen
Galactorrhoea	fluid in the breast when not breast feeding
Glaucoma	disease of the eye characterized by raised pressure in the eyeball
Glucose	a form of sugar found in the blood
Gonadotrophin	hormone produced by the pituitary acting on the gonads, either testes or ovary
Gynaecology	study of the diseases of women
Haemorrhage	loss of blood, bleeding
Hormones	chemicals, produced by the glands, which exert an action at a distant site
Hyperglycaemia	raised blood sugar
Hypoglycaemia	lowered blood sugar
Hypothalamus	specialized part of the brain concerned with control of body functions
Implant	pellet of drug inserted into the tissues
Intermenstruum	part of the menstrual cycle not covered by the premenstruum or menstruation,

	usually days 5 to 24
Inter-uterine device	small contraceptive appliance inserted into the womb
Labour	birth of baby
Lactation	breast feeding
Lethargy	excessive tiredness
Libido	sex drive
Luteinizing hormone	hormone produced by the pituitary which causes ovulation and the production of progesterone
Menarche	first menstruation
Menopause	last menstruation, marking the end of the childbearing years
Menstrual clock	specialized portion of the hypothalamus responsible for the cyclical timing of menstruation
Menstrual cycle	time from first day of menstruation until the first day of the next menstruation
Menstrual loss	bleeding at menstruation
Menstruation	monthly bleeding from the vagina in women of childbearing age
Metabolism	building up and breaking down of chemicals in the body
Migraine	severe form of headache
Mittelschmerz	abdominal pain accompanying ovulation
Oestrogen	hormone released by the ovary
Ovary	reproductive organ containing egg cells
Ovulation	release of egg cell from the ovary
Ovum	egg cell
Paramenstruum	premenstruum and menstruation
Pituitary	gland situated at the base of the brain and controlling many other glands

Placebo	inactive or inert substance with no curative value
Placenta	organ which develops within the womb responsible for feeding the foetus and for the production of the hormones of pregnancy
Postmenstruum	the days immediately after menstruation
Postnatal	after childbirth
Potassium	mineral present in blood and cells of the body
Premenstruum	the days immediately prior to menstruation
Preovulatory	the days immediately before ovulation
Progesterone	hormone produced by the ovaries, adrenals and by the placenta during pregnancy
Progestogen	man-made drug used for contraception, which was once thought to be a substitute for natural progesterone
Prolactin	hormone produced by the pituitary gland
Puerperium	time after childbirth
Pyridoxine	vitamin B6
Sodium	mineral present in the blood and cells of the body
Spasmodic	coming in spasms
Sterilization	operation to prevent conception permanently
Synchrony	at the same time
Syndrome	collection of symptoms which commonly occur together
Testosterone	male hormone
Therapy	treatment
Trauma	injury

Uterus	womb
Vagina	passage leading from the exterior of the body to the mouth of the womb

Index